Conversations with my Son

A Diary

TerryAnn Fisher
and Troy Michaels

iUniverse, Inc.
New York Bloomington

Conversations with my Son
A Diary

iUniverse books may be ordered through booksellers or by contacting:

iUniverse
1663 Liberty Drive
Bloomington, IN 47403
www.iuniverse.com
1-800-Authors (1-800-288-4677)

Because of the dynamic nature of the Internet, any Web addresses or links contained in this book may have changed since publication and may no longer be valid.

ISBN: 978-1-4502-2997-5 (sc)
ISBN: 978-1-4502-3002-5 (dj)
ISBN: 978-1-4502-2998-2 (ebk)

Library of Congress Control Number: 2010906380

Printed in the United States of America

iUniverse rev. date: 8/24/2010

A Letter From Troy

So, Mother,

Am sending you an unusual letter. Am sending you my Living Will or a copy of one. And a copy of the doctor's business card. I want you to consult with him if there is any reason I am unconscious. "Life sustaining" would mean that the physical body is not able to function on its own and without whatever mechanical apparatus or device. I see no need to have one hooked to my body. There may be a need for a breathing machine, but if I cannot breathe on my own, *no way*. Again, if the physical body is in a state that does not function on its own, forget it.

But do seek consultation with the doctor, and think about what he says.

I do not want to distress you or any of that, but as I do have AIDS, it's important to discuss and think about this now rather than later. Even though I will have talked to you by the time you get this, I am still sending you my thoughts.

I did see the doctor yesterday (It's now December 4, 12:30 AM, just past midnight), and I really like him. Feel he's a good doctor. He did say that I am showing signs of things that naturally occur with people who have AIDS, so it made me feel better to know what's happening.

Right now they are just little things, like the "Itchy Bump Disease", drying skin, and diarrhea. When I see the other doctor, he'll send off a stool sample (no joke from me) to see why I'm experiencing diarrhea. So I'll also just live and do things to be healthy.

Otherwise not much else to say; just what I told you as I feel it's important and again better now than never or later.

Know that I love you and remember our agreement to meet again on the higher planes of God, to discuss our connection, where and why it all started, etc., etc.

Again, love you and am grateful for times we've shared. Boo hoo. Boo hoo. Lovely sentiments. But like you told me, I'd rather have you know as not to.

Oh. Why did I choose to come to stay with you in the future rather than with Dad? Well, you and I have talked a lot about death and dying, about what our thoughts and views are. Right now, Dad is not ready to talk about these things. So that's why.

So anything else to say? Boo hoo. Yes, allow me to go when it's my time. If you are there when the translation happens for me, do this for me: Give me a hug. Allow the love we share to open your heart, and in that love sing a chant for me and tell me that (my religious leader) will be there to guide me across. But do allow me to go. Boo hoo. What a sad letter … or what? Boo hoo. Boo hoo.

So that's all, and I haven't translated/died yet. So let's just keep it in the background.

Love,

Your son, Troy

Chapter 1

Sunday October 11 (the following year)

I need to vent and get past all that's happened this summer so that I can move on.

I'm sure I'm going to find this to be dull reading someday, but, then, what's a diary to be ? For me, right now, it's an outlet for the stress that I am able, finally, to see at a distance.

It's been a traumatic summer. Now I have some spare time and the chance to write down what happened so I can put it behind me. I'd like to be objective and look toward the future.

First, a happy thought: in a few days, David and I will have been married fourteen years. Perhaps now we can look forward to being quietly together.

When we moved here a few years ago, we really did, oddly, believe that our lives would continue in the same way they did at the Grand Canyon: we'd continue to go to work every day, come home at night, spend time together, and get up and do it again. It just didn't turn out that way this year.

Mom and Dad came to visit in early June. What was going to be a short, happy trip turned out to a much longer, uncomfortable stay for them when Mom slipped and broke her right hip during a sightseeing trip to a small town south of here.

Dad slipped and fell twice at the motel where he was staying next to the hospital but, fortunately, suffered only a sprained ankle.

While Mom was in the hospital, I was laid off from my security job at State University. More city police officers were brought on campus. The last seven security officers hired were given a choice of going to the custodial department or getting unemployment. I chose unemployment.

I wonder how many other people have moved someplace thinking that the job they moved for would last forever. It does help, actually, knowing that I'm not the only person who has done that, but it doesn't change my mind about wanting another job as soon as possible.

After Mom had recuperated enough to fly back to Arizona, she and Dad had to wait all day in the airport for a bigger plane to arrive. It turned out that, even though I had been told by the airline that she would not have trouble getting onto the plane, there was no lift available for her original flight and she could not climb the stairs.

There was a highlight, though … Troy came to visit in August.

Although he looked tired and thin, he seemed to walk easily from the airport arrival gate to the car. He has always enjoyed flying, so I think it was a treat for him to be able to come for a visit.

He brought me a tea set of a mother rabbit for the teapot and two baby rabbits, one for sugar and one for milk. All are black and white and so cute. He said that he had seen them in tea set shop and "heard them calling his name", so he bought them for me. He had a nice smile with that statement. Thank goodness he has a sense of humor!

One day we went to the big mall in town and he bought me a Pocket Dragon. Its name is actually "Stalking the Cookie Jar", but I'll call it Cookie. I put it on the window sill in front of the sink.

One evening the two of us went to a mystery dinner theatre. It was held in one of the historic houses in town. The house had a big porch on the front where we had dinner after the mystery tour throughout the house. Although Troy and I were members in the audience, we were incorporated into the production as Mr. Holmes and Dr. Watson. Troy was asked to give a speech at dinner as Mr. Holmes. We were both surprised. The lady across from me leaned toward me and asked if we were actually members of the play. I said no. The dinner is such a nice memory after having been upset the rest of the summer.

Troy stayed for about two weeks.

So today I am remembering those good and sad memories.

Monday October 12

It seems that maybe it really will be fall, my favorite season. It's another day of cool, fresh air.

Here I am, now sitting at the picnic table in our front yard with a glass of tea by my pad. I can sit quietly and write and enjoy the weather. There is something about fall that gives me a strange pleasant, grounded type of feeling. Fall lets me know that life is the same, season after season, with the regularity of life in general. In a strange way, it makes me feel safe. I don't know if it's the soft sound of falling leaves hitting the ground, the crisp smell, or just what it is, but there is definitely something comforting about the season, even if I can't identify it.

We have typical Midwest weather here, not as pretty as in the East or in the Western mountain areas. The colors are subtle and rather muddy looking because of the more moderate temperatures which don't seem to change much. There are still muted yellow, red, and orange leaves, though, so we do get to see some bright fall color.

Our yard tends toward green until the leaves slowly change color here and there. When the leaves finally fall the branches begin to look stark against the sky.

But the feel and clean smell is definitely fall, letting us know that winter will be arriving before long.

It's been a busy day so far. I went to the post office to mail more résumés and to the bank and to town to fill out a job application at the hospital for a receptionist position. I took a typing test at another place, ate lunch at the diner downtown, and *finally* came home. Rushing from place to place is probably going to be the story of my life for a while, though I can only hope that things will become better than they have been this year so far.

While I've been sitting here, a large flock of medium-sized black birds has flown down from the north. They're sitting in the trees, squawking and yelling to each other. Suddenly they'll be gone, migrating someplace else. It reminds me of an Indian belief that when a large flock of birds arrives, something bad is happening or going to happen. So far today everything seems fine; except now there's the somewhat eerie feeling of Hitchcock's movie.

My father called a couple nights ago and said that while he was lifting my mother's wheelchair into the car, one of the steel rods he had to have put into his back several years ago had broken. He will have to have the rod replaced. A friend took him to the doctor, who made an appointment for the operation on October 23. I'd like to visit them after they find out what will happen if Daddy needs to go for a long stay in the hospital. Mother will need rides to Tucson.

Troy called last night about his visit to his father and sister. He said that he had a good time, but that he was so exhausted while he was in the St. Louis airport that he forgot whether he was going *to* Ohio or coming *from* Ohio. He ended up missing his plane to Chicago. Also, he was having trouble breathing. The airline provided him with a wheelchair, though, and rescheduled him on a flight an hour later. After telling me all that he said he thinks I'm relaxed and easygoing and that it is easy to talk to me. I think that little does he know that all I want to do is scream, "I can't handle this!"

I remember when he called me at the Grand Canyon years ago and told me he had AIDS. I couldn't believe it and wouldn't admit that he would be dying someday, possibly even before me. He said he found out when he had applied for the Coast Guard and had to take a blood test. I can only hope that the recruiter was kind and sensitive when he told Troy that he had the virus.

Troy's sister, Teresa, called and said that she and her father have ordered Troy some expedition-type long underwear. It's back-ordered, though. They were upset about how he looked when he visited and said I hadn't warned them enough. I had told them that he was sick, but I guess I didn't stress how sick he *looks*. Did I not notice when he visited us in August? Have I been denying how sick he really is?

I seem to just be going on and on. I wonder if I'm going to want to keep this to remember what has happened this summer or throw it away so I can just *forget!* I ask myself, who else can I "write" to? I can't complain to David or my friends about the same thing all the time!

Tuesday October 13

I went to town today and bought Troy a pair of really cute brown and white St. Bernard dog slippers, some mixed-wool socks, and a couple pairs of long underwear. I'll mail everything tomorrow so he'll have it to use while he's waiting for the back-ordered long underwear from Teresa and their father. It's cold in his apartment.

Thursday October 15

The man who was director of the AIDS Project when I started volunteering there several years ago died yesterday. His memorial service is today, but I don't think I'll go.

It's 3:51 PM and beautiful, beautiful out. But there are dark clouds in the south. Between all the black birds the other day and all the clouds today I wonder what that means. I am probably being superstitious. So there are birds and clouds. Aren't there "always" ?! I'm sure I'm being silly and am probably depressed since I don't have a job right now.

A year ago today, I was on my way to Chicago to visit Troy. I took a bus and a train. I really enjoyed the train ride. The bus ride was just long and cramped.

Chapter 2

Troy is in the hospital!!!

He's been there since yesterday but didn't call me. I found out when I called his apartment tonight, and J, the fellow he shares the apartment with, answered the phone and told me. I had called J, actually, rather than Troy since I'd been concerned about him since the St. Louis Airport incident. I didn't want him to think I'm over-mothering him, though. I wanted J's opinion about whether or not I should encourage Troy to quit work. He's worked every day; no disability insurance, no staying home. It's quite an accomplishment for someone who has been as sick apparently as he must have been getting.

I thought I could suggest that Troy might want to come here or go to Dayton to rest and maybe volunteer a little. I could look into some financial help here so he wouldn't feel dependent. I guess that now it's not something that he will need to think about until he gets out of the hospital. We can see how he feels then and what he wants to do.

Troy has Kaposi's of the mouth and lungs, plus some kind of pneumonia. He's in the hospital so he can have some kind of tests done.

Saturday October 17

Troy called earlier this morning to let me know how he is. He didn't sound as if he is concerned about being in the hospital. He acted as if this is just something that the doctor wanted to do to monitor him.

It's David's and my fourteenth wedding anniversary. We hadn't planned on doing anything particular or exciting. Last week, we did talk about maybe going out to eat tonight or to see a movie tomorrow. In Arizona we would probably have gone to Prescott or maybe even to Laughlin. Right now, though, I'd prefer to just stay home and wait for another call from Troy.

How can I stay here right now, though, and not get up and go to Chicago and see what's happening?

Maybe I just can't admit that Troy is as sick as he may be and want to wait until he calls me to tell me to come up.

I could apply for unemployment there and look for a temporary job and be there till he gets better. It is so difficult to think clearly and to make what seem to be rational decisions.

Later …

Troy called me about 9:30 PM and asked if I was sitting down. He is being taken to Intensive Care because he's not getting enough oxygen in his blood. Visiting hours are for fifteen minutes, every two hours.

Chapter 3

I've taken a train to Chicago after a bus ride to St. Louis. I love trains, but it's really sad that this time the reason was not for pleasure. The sound and the rolling motion, which is usually so nice, just kept seeming to say, "Let's go faster. Let's go faster."

I took a cab to Troy's apartment. I could have taken the El but felt that I would be too confused and would be wasting my time trying to find my way around. I can take the El into the city when I leave, but that may be a long time from now. Obviously, I don't know what I'm going to be doing or what is going to be happening. I can't plan ahead yet.

I like Chicago. It seems like a small town to me even though I don't know how to get everywhere yet. Fortunately, visiting last year helped since Troy and I walked around his neighborhood and downtown and went to Chinatown, where we had lunch. So I have some idea of where I am. I was even able to tell the cab driver where we needed to turn when he couldn't find the street. It is such a sad trip this time without Troy to meet me at the train and laugh when we're together.

When I left last year to come home, we got off the El and walked a little down the street before Troy said to stop. He moved off the sidewalk to the street and waved down a cab. It was like being in a movie.

On the way to the hospital I asked a police officer for directions. He kept giving me intersection information or something. Turns out that Chicago uses block number intersection directions or something like that. I just didn't understand. All I wanted to do was cry. It's very confusing if you don't know where the streets are to begin with. I guess I haven't lived here long enough to understand what I was being told.

I kept walking and finally found an El station. Sitting in what looked like a phone booth in the dark shade of the El was a ticket issuer, who gave me directions on where to get off and on the El. He even told me welcome to Chicago!

I finally found the hospital and visited Troy. I'm sure he must be scared, but I didn't ask him. He's always been thin but seems even thinner than he was when he visited David and me in August, if that's possible. He doesn't know how long he'll be in the hospital.

There is so much to think about what to do. I think I will be staying here in town for awhile. I will need to check in with unemployment on a courtesy claim about getting a job here. I'll also need to see about getting Home Health to stay with Troy while I work. He can rest and then decide if he wants to live with David and me or go to Ohio to stay with Teresa and his dad. I can't imagine that he's strong enough to go back to work.

Chapter 4

Monday October 19

Troy was moved from Intensive Care to a big sunny room on a regular nursing floor since he's doing better. But about 11:30 tonight he called the apartment and asked J to bring me to the hospital *right away*!!!

He'd had a panic attack when he was coming out of the bathroom. The oxygen meter came off his thumb and was making the loud noise it does when not attached. He said he kept thinking, "I'm alive!" but the machine kept beeping and beeping and beeping. I offered to stay all night (he has a private room), but he said he'd be all right now that he knows how the meter works.

Tuesday October 20

I visited with Troy, and we just generally hung out. Well, as much as people can do in a hospital when one of them is a patient. He looks okay, and the nurses are keeping an eye on his breathing.

Although it is not that far from the hospital by bus, it's a long, lonely trip back to the apartment.

Chapter 5

Wednesday October 21

8:30 AM

I'm going to go to the unemployment office today. One of Troy's friends will take me over since I don't know where it is. I'll take the bus back to the hospital.

I am so scared, though!!! Unless I get back to my normal reactions, the agents at the unemployment office are going to think I'm on drugs!!!

I called Troy rather than going to the hospital first. He said rather stiffly to call back this afternoon.

Evening ...

The unemployment agent was very helpful. Both the agent and the man at the El station were so nice to me. It's like they cared even though they don't know me.

I will stay all night at the hospital tonight. Just before I got ready to leave, Troy asked if I would stay, so I'll sleep in his room on some chairs pushed together.

Chapter 6

Thursday October 22

It's Mom and Dad's 60th anniversary.

Since I stayed in the hospital last night, I went back to the apartment a while ago to pick up some clothes. Staying with Troy will be much more comfortable than *trying* to sleep at his apartment. All I do is worry.

I'm glad I stayed last night. It seemed like Troy's oxygen alarm went off all the time. He would relax and his breathing would slow down, and the alarm would go off. At least I was there to talk to him and reassure him that he was okay and still alive.

Also, one of the doctors gave him a "mild" sleeping pill that he *really* reacted badly to. He got out of bed and started walking to the bathroom talking about the people having a party in the room. It was scary. I don't think he'll be taking any more sleeping pills.

I went into The City today and made some job contacts. It was my first El ride downtown by myself. It was a lot easier than I thought it would be trying to find the way around alone. Of course having Troy show me around last year really helped.

When I got downtown, I went into the building where Troy's company's personnel office is. I called Troy to tell him I had made it downtown okay on my own. To a small town woman, entering the lobby was like walking into a movie set. It was a big, Art Deco-styled space with high, carved ceilings. The walls were honey-colored marble of an almost amber shade. I could imagine someone hurrying across the lobby to the phones on the far wall to make a call. This time it was me.

I hurried from building to building and office to office pretending that Troy and I were together and he was telling me about where "we" were.

After I had dropped off my résumés at several businesses and was on my way back to the hospital, I stopped at a Buddhist temple I had found on one of my walks to the hospital from the bus the other day. The temple is only about a block and a half from the hospital. A short, round, very nice monk showed me to a small garden where I sat and tried to be quiet for awhile. The garden had pots of plants and lots of tile on the ground but not much grass. There was some city noise, but what there was sounded far in the distance. It was very peaceful.

Chapter 7

Friday October 23

The post office sent a notice that the dog slippers I had sent to Troy had arrived, so I went to pick them up. It's one of those days when it's too warm to wear a jacket, so I began to sweat. I took off my jacket, and then the wind blew and I got cold. There were no cabs or buses to catch in the area, so all I could do was just walk. I wish I had thought to bring my vest with me.

When I got to the hospital, I was chilled and felt like I was getting sick. I stopped at the nurses' desk to ask for a face mask so I won't be kept out of Troy's room.

I also stopped again at the Buddhist temple on the way to the hospital after picking up the package. Maybe I can go to the services there sometimes.

Today was Troy's first good day. He said, "I feel like I'm alive."

Chapter 8

I called Mom and Dad today to tell them happy anniversary, since I wanted to wait and see what Dad's doctor said. He'll have an operation on the broken rod on December 1. They still plan to live there rather than move near David and me.

Troy's doctor said Troy can leave the hospital next week.

I saw this on one of the signs inside the bus yesterday:

I have always known
That at last I would
Take this road, but yesterday
I did not know it would be today.
—Ariwara no Narihira 9th Century Japan

Chapter 9

Sunday October 25

Troy is not feeling good today. His temperature is up to 100.4. He is talking again about maybe not leaving the hospital. His appetite is gone because of the thrush in his mouth, so he can't taste food very well.

Tonight I will sleep on the other bed in Troy's room … I've been sleeping on three armless chairs pushed together to make a sort of flat surface. Troy said that since he is in isolation I should just sleep in the empty bed.

I went to the small hospital dining room again for dinner tonight. It is a pleasant and nicely decorated area that makes it seem like life is normal. Sitting in there is like being in a restaurant. There is no noisiness and clatter like in the bigger room where most of the nursing personnel sit finally having a chance to talk to each other.

I sat there eating and trying to read instead of jumping up and screaming, "My son is sick and has a terminal illness!" How can I even say the word "dying" out loud to other people when I usually can't even say it to myself?!

When I came back from dinner, Troy said he will be using oxygen awhile to see how it feels and if it helps him.

I sat and looked out the window to the apartment building across the street. It is brick in an upside down U-shape from where I sit. I can see that it is four storeys tall with grass between the sidewalks that

16

branch into each section. There is an old-fashioned fountain where the sidewalks meet. People are actually having real lives in there. I guess this is our real life right now, though it's very difficult to feel that anything like this is real. I guess I just won't let myself believe it.

Monday October 26

Troy's temperature is down to 98.8.

I went into the city again to apply for a job. I'm applying at one of the women's centers. That would be nice. I think I'd like working someplace like that. I could get Troy some help with visiting nurses during the day and be home with him at night.

I've spent over $300 so far for the El, buses, taxi fares, and food. How could I have spent that much so quickly? I've been here only eight days!

Troy's doctor said that they'll still use oxygen but it will be down to 3 liters instead of 6, and they'll see how that is.

I lie in my bed at night, the light shining in from the street lights below, and wonder if Troy is scared. I don't ask, though. Maybe I need to ask about more things than I do, but I am afraid of what his answer will be. Maybe I'm not much help to him.

The fear takes me, and I feel like Scarlett O'Hara in *Gone With The Wind*: I'll think about it tomorrow.

Tuesday October 27

What makes stress? Let me count the ways.

The *good* stress is that it looks like Troy can go home tomorrow. But he has not urinated much today even though he's drinking water. The *bad* stress is that I've got only $180 left. More *bad* stress: I think that I mailed my courtesy unemployment form to the wrong office. Maybe I can go in to the unemployment office and pick up two more. That's *good* stress—something I can take care of.

Chapter 10

Troy is back in his apartment. A fellow he knows came over and took me to the unemployment office to get the paperwork during Troy's lunchtime. Afterward, we got some lunch together and then drove to the hospital. We had to park about three blocks from the hospital and walk over to find out what time Troy would get out. Even though it was chilly, it was sunny.

Troy got here about 2:00 or 3:00 in the afternoon.

His apartment is on the third floor. Since there is no elevator, he would climb a few steps and then sit down. He "sat" his way up each step because he is so tired. I wish I were strong enough to carry him.

He said that he might continue to work at his job till spring and then leave. Later, he said that maybe he'd work till the end of November. Finally he said he might quit work and not go back. If he quit, he could stay here until I could come back and pick him up after he's rested. That way I can go home first and come and get him later. We could see if he could get Home Health to come in and check on him regularly.

We had chili and green beans for dinner and got to bed about 6:00 PM.

When I got up to go into the bathroom about 7:00, J said that David had called. I called him back but was so tired I could barely talk.

18

I told him that Troy was back in the apartment but we didn't know yet what we were going to do.

Thursday October 29

It's 11:30 AM. We slept till about 8:30. Tim said he'd like to go back with me. He's just too cold here. It's a relief that he is considering not staying here. It might be different if it were summer, but now winter is coming and he will just be too uncomfortable. I'll see about renting a van and leaving the weekend after this. That way he can see his doctor here next week before we leave.

Friday October 30

12:20 PM

I've spent all morning calling doctors near my house, and now I'm waiting for callbacks. One doctor can't take Troy until after Thanksgiving. Maybe the AIDS Project can help. I'm trying to … I don't know what I'm trying to do. Maybe it's just wait patiently (me?!) and hope that once we move and get settled Troy will get "better". He says he'll use a walker there. It'll give him more mobility around the house.

Now all that remains today is to try to sit patiently, appear calm, and act like everything is natural and okay so that Troy is not upset more than he needs to be.

Saturday October 31

Lying in bed this morning I was freaking out about all that has to be done. Then I finally decided that all I could concentrate on was doing the wash. Troy's friends can help him pack. One of them came over and drove me to the laundromat and back. They are being so helpful!

A family who are friends of his came over to visit on their way to a party. They are really neat people. They're all individuals with their own interests and outlooks and are very loving toward each other. They're very different from people who seem to want their family members to be clones of themselves.

After the family left, Troy, his friends who weren't going to the party, and I had our own party, with pizza.

Troy says maybe I'm learning about priorities and letting go. I don't know about that.

Sunday November 1

Troy's lesson: I told him this morning about learning what his responsibility is for himself now that he's sick. We lay around the apartment and talked about the karma we have together to work through as a team. David probably fits in there someplace, too, I'm sure, but I don't know where yet. All this is very "interesting," though so sad. I am trying to keep the word "sad" out of my vocabulary, although it seems like the word still stays there.

Thinking about the trip home is somewhat scary. Will Troy survive? Won't he? What will happen on the way? Will he be comfortable? If he gets sicker, will there be a hospital and doctors near where we are?

I've bought an egg crate mattress to cut down to fit comfortably on the front seat so he can lie down if he wants to. Maybe that will be more comfortable for him than having to sit up all the time.

As the time gets closer I like to think that I'm more relaxed about details; then I'm overwhelmed again. I try to tell myself that things will get done, and we'll leave, and we'll deal with the future as it unfolds. Nervous though I am about it, maybe it helps to remember that, each in our own way, we're doing this together.

Monday November 2

I'm stressed out again. It's because of the waiting for Troy's company's insurance paperwork to be taken care of. It has to be changed over to private insurance so Troy will be covered when he leaves the state.

David says to relax; we have to take our time. We have *one* chance to get the best insurance benefits for Troy that we can.

I upset Troy by being upset myself, but I don't know how to help it.

One of his friends said that layoff is a crock and total disability is better. Another said to call a lawyer for advice.

Tuesday November 3

I couldn't sleep last night even though Troy gave me one of his muscle relaxants. I guess it wore off. All I could think about was that I'm not feeding him enough.

I also walked to the bus stop and took a bus to the Sears store to get him some long underwear pants. Apparently the ones Teresa sent were lost in transit someplace. Sears is on the road to Cicero. It's odd, thinking that I'm in the same town where Al Capone used to live. I also got Troy two sweat suits—one red and one blue. Hopefully those will help keep him warm.

I've decided to make my goal to try to feed Troy while all the exterior stuff swirls around us. Maybe we can make a little hollow for us to be "safe" in.

5:15 PM

AIDS legal counsel called to say that Troy is protected no matter what, but the best insurance would be private insurance.

Wednesday November 4

Another day of waiting to find out about what will happen about Troy's insurance. Maybe we can get a lawyer here so I can go to into the city Friday morning and sign the papers and we can leave this weekend.

Thursday November 5

Busy day!!!

First I went to town to see the company's medical liaison to pick up papers for Troy to sign for health insurance. Then I took Troy to the doctor, who said that he can travel. When we got back to the apartment, Troy "sat" up the stairs again, one step at a time. When we got to the second floor he lay down over several steps to rest. Then got up to go into an apartment. I told him we had another flight to go. "Silly me," he said. He hadn't counted enough flights. It was so sad.

Then I went back downtown to take the insurance forms and medical records to the liaison.

I looked out the El windows and remembered the times Troy and I rode it, and now I realize that we will probably never ride it together again. I'll remember the buildings and the horse barn where the carriage horses are kept. I took a picture of the statue of the couple climbing up the outside of one of the buildings trying to get to an office inside. Troy told me last year that this was an ad that was put up when the building opened but was never taken down.

I thought about one of our rides into town then: Troy was pointing out different places along the way. A teenage girl behind us was making fun of us. I felt sorry for her. We can see a city any day on television that looks like where she lives, but what does she know about long vistas of hills in the distance or being able to see big puffy clouds overhead that aren't obscured by dark buildings. She will probably never see the Grand Canyon or a national park or beauty beyond a small park or a zoo. The air she breathes will probably always have a hint of exhaust. There will be car noise all night long, not the quiet with the melodic call of frogs or an occasional bird chirp. Days will have honking and people yelling, not cows mooing in the distance.

My father is having his back operation this Monday. It seems the rod has slipped through the skin. Mom is hoping he can get a private room so she can stay with him and won't have to worry about how to get back and forth to see him. She can't drive anymore and otherwise will have to depend on friends. The hospital is over twenty-five miles from their house. I sure do wish they'd move near David and me. Even with Troy sick I could still help them out if they were living near us.

Friday November 6

Troy's taste buds are going bad again. We're hoping the doctor can give him medicine for thrush or whatever his problem is.

I'll pick up the moving truck tomorrow, and his friends will come over to help move. Then maybe we can get out of here.

He said that he will have to learn to look at life from a new angle now.

I called State University to find out about work gossip. My old nine-month position is open, but the lady who has seniority over the rest of us who were laid off will probably take it, even though she now has a twelve-month custodial position. I have mixed feelings, though now I'm glad I took the layoff choice instead of the offered janitor position. I would not have done a good job as janitor. Even though I haven't found a regular job yet, I feel like I'm doing better than if I were to end up with a bad job reputation. At least I'm on the rehire list until July.

One of my favorite memories of working on campus at night is of the air crystallizing. I'm not sure just what happened, perhaps it was due to the humidity in the air when it was cold enough to freeze. I could see what looked like little falling "jewels" when I got to a lighted area along the sidewalk. This did not seem to happen frequently, so it was always a pleasant surprise when it did.

Chapter 11

Saturday November 7

I picked up the moving truck today. Troy's friends and I carried his stuff down the typical narrow steps with tight corners shown in the comedies with people getting stuck with a large couch. But we got everything into the truck. Troy actually doesn't have too much. He's moved to so many different cities that he hasn't acquired a lot, or at least he hasn't acquired a lot of *big* things.

Sherry, another friend of Troy's, came over and sat with him while the rest of us were running around. Although I'd talked to her on the phone I'd never met her before. She seems nice. After she left he said sadly, "If things had been different …"

He's had several girlfriends, including a longtime girlfriend when he was at school, but they realized that a life together wouldn't work out. Sometimes things just aren't "meant to be" between people for whatever reason.

Sunday November 8

It's a quiet day. We're resting up for the trip. We'll start tomorrow. I'm both anxious and reluctant to get started. Troy is tired. I haven't asked him if he's scared.

Chapter 12

Monday November 9

We didn't leave till early afternoon. We made it to Bloomington and are staying at a motel across the street from a restaurant. Traffic is heavy, so I have to drive the truck over and back with food. Troy said that he wanted to stay in the room. He couldn't rest very well on the trip here. There wasn't any room to stretch out, of course, so he put his head on my lap. I don't imagine he could sleep well either with the steering wheel in his face. I bought a cheeseburger for him and a big salad for me. I am going to take the trip slowly so we don't get overtired.

Tuesday November 10

We got to St. Louis and drove across town so we don't have to worry about getting stuck in traffic tomorrow morning when we leave. Again, there's a nearby restaurant. This time it's on the same side of the street as our motel, though, so I walked over and back with dinner.

Troy is staying in the room and not coming with me when I go out to get food. I keep remembering times when we would go out and take long walks together. I wonder if we appreciated that enough.

Chapter 13

Wednesday November 11

Well, we made it home. I will be unloading the truck, but not right away. It's all too much without a rest first.

Also, by using rubber gloves and a little common sense and caution, unless things get worse I think Troy will be very easy to take care of.

At least we're here and warm.

We'll rest now.

Thursday November 12

I'm sleeping in my room, and Troy is in the guest room that faces the outside of the house. When I went in to check on him in the middle of the night, I heard a frog croaking outside his window. It rained all night and early morning.

Friday November 13

The visiting nurse was here today. It's arranged that Troy can get coverage and be in the Home Health Program.

Sherry, who visited Troy in Chicago, sent flowers. I'll pick them up tomorrow.

Troy's also received a large card and several small handmade cards from some of the people he worked with. It is so nice that he's remembered by so many people.

Saturday November 14

Troy's temperature was 101.6 at 1:55 this morning. I called the visiting nurse. It hovered at about 100+ till about 6:45 AM when it was 99.2. I had made up my mind to take him to the doctor if it was still high by 10:00 AM, but by then it was down to 97.8.

We're having a new septic tank pipe put in. It will be done soon. We can still use the toilet connected to the old one in the meantime, though. Someday maybe the small town we live near will have a sewer system and we'll be hooked up to it. Not yet, though.

The flowers Sherry sent are dark red carnations, white mums, yellow daisies, and purple "somethings" in a gold pot. Troy said carnations are his favorite flower. These smell only faintly and don't have the spicy scent he likes, though. But they are very pretty. It is so nice of her.

Today is Teresa's birthday.

Chapter 14

I took Troy to the Emergency Room late last night. His temperature was 100+ again and he hadn't been urinating, so I called the Visiting Nurses. Of course I thought of renal failure. The nurse said to take him in, so I did. I expected to either have him admitted or for it to take "forever" since it was a Saturday night. But maybe it wasn't busy since it's starting to get cold out.

He was catheterized without much urine retention, so we left and got home about midnight.

I saw his bedsore, which I hadn't seen before. We didn't even know he had one. It is at the end of his tailbone and about an inch or two long and a half inch wide.

Chapter 15

Troy and I cried together for the first time.

When he was showering, he found what he thinks are Kaposi marks. He is afraid of possible pain and turning purple. We hugged each other and cried. I told him I don't care what color he is and that we'll get medication for his pain. I'm *so* glad he is here!

He says that he thinks it's better that he's staying here with us since his dad's house has two floors. I don't know if he could get up and down the stairs. He would have to stay upstairs all the time rather than downstairs "where the action is" since the bathroom is up there.

My house is an earth berm: one floor with dirt piled to the edge of the roof on three sides. We have a woodstove, and it's a little easier to heat. The bathroom has the toilet in a little alcove, and Troy can sit sideways and lean on a wall if it's too painful for him to sit up straight.

I know it was difficult for him to decide where he wanted to be. Also, maybe he thinks his father couldn't handle this. I'm not even sure if I can, but I will certainly not express that thought to him!

Tuesday November 17

Sometime in the middle of the night Troy called me and said he was "back again". For a while, he said, he had been dead, although he couldn't explain exactly what he meant.

After David left for work, I went into his bedroom and lay in bed with him, and we cried some more. He screamed his frustration: "I don't want to die!"

We went to the doctor this morning, who said that Troy's bedsore may actually be herpes and prescribed medication. It's expensive, but if it works and makes Troy more comfortable, it will be worth it.

Troy acted very peculiar on the way to and from the doctor. It was very scary since it was like his mind was leaving. He asked the same questions in a rhythmic way over and over and over all the way there and back: "Where are we going? When will we get there? What will we do? Where are we going? When will we get there? What will we do?" I tried to answer him calmly each time, trying not to upset him as much as I was upset or to let him know he was repeating himself. He seemed to be regressing/forgetting.

I didn't know what to do. I stopped at the store and bought some of the perfume that I had worn when he was growing up. I locked the car doors when I went inside so he couldn't open any and get out, even though I don't think he could walk far.

When we got home I got out the small scrapbooks I've kept with pictures of him, his sisters, my parents and grandmother. We sat together and looked through them, and he told me who everybody was. He looked at pictures of himself when he was younger and said, sadly and quietly, "I was nice looking, wasn't I? The kids used to make fun of me, though, at school."

Maybe the stress of going to the doctor upset him, since he hasn't been like that when we've been at home. It was frightening. If it happens again, how can I allow him to go into a nursing home and see him only occasionally?

He doesn't remember his trip to his father's house in October or being in the hospital in Chicago. He said that the trip we'd just come back from to the doctor was beginning to blur. He kept apologizing and said several times, "I'm sorry, but I'm a little disoriented."

He told me that he told himself this morning that he is really going to die and that it was the first time he admitted it to himself.

Our friends from out of town called and asked about loaning us their wheelchair. They'll bring it Monday. It will be helpful. Perhaps we'll be able to go the Mall and I can push him around or we can go to the grocery or ??? … just get outside sometimes so life seems somewhat natural to him?

Wednesday November 18

It's a scary, awful, terribly frightening time. I can't tell if Troy is having an extreme reaction to his new medication or just what. Yesterday he seemed to be deteriorating mentally. All I can do is sit and be quiet and try to be calm for him.

At 11:30 last night I helped him to the bathroom. When I walked him in there, he had begun getting a skeletal look. By the time he got back to bed, he had dark, shrunken areas around his eyes, or I would have thought he was trying to play a joke when he began asking questions. He could not remember how he got here, how he'd gotten to the hospital in Chicago, or who other people were. One time he referred to David as Mr. Fisher. He said over and over in the middle of conversations, "I have AIDS. It's Acquired Immune Deficiency Syndrome. What's AIDS? Is it a homosexual disease? Am I a homosexual?" He asked about bowel movements and how could he tell he was going to have one. Why does he have to sit sideways on the toilet?

I went back into the bathroom to flush the toilet, and when I walked back into his bedroom he looked startled and did not know who I was. I tried again to patiently and calmly answer the questions he asked. I could only scream inside "*No!* This can't be real! He *has to be* kidding me, pretending, trying to fool me, so that later we can laugh about it!" But I knew he *wasn't* kidding and that this horrible episode was as real as any "normal" aspect of his experience.

He was hollow-eyed, flailing the air like a baby bird trying to fly. This was *not* someone trying to be funny! He survived the episode yesterday, but there could be many more, each individually as terrifying as that one and this one have been. It has seemed as if I have been watching his brain literally short-circuit.

He was very agitated.

We locked the front door so he won't wander off.

I gave him some medication today at 1:45 PM and then again at 5:00 PM, although I skipped 8:00 PM so I can begin a new series of doses tomorrow. I was sure it was a reaction to the medication and called the Osco Drug hotline to find out definite side effects.

The confusion happened so quickly, except for the first questions yesterday, that it made me wonder if he is beginning to have mental problems.

Thursday November 19

About 3:00 AM I went into Troy's room to see how he was. He was himself again. It makes me wonder how *I* will be if he gets "bad" permanently. I would have called the doctor this morning if he hadn't improved, but what will happen if this happens again and he *doesn't* get better that time? What if he needs to be put into a nursing home because of his mental deterioration? Could the problem be an infection and not the medication?

He said when I went into his room that he remembered the whole episode but that there was nothing he could do about it at the time. He also remembered all the things that he'd forgotten earlier. It was one of the most awful experiences of my life. He seemed calm, though, when he was telling me about it. But imagine how the relatives of people with Alzheimer's must feel. *That* is permanent.

Troy seems to be over the episode.

Over the years, Troy has slowly changed parts of his name trying to "find himself," as it used to be called in the sixties and seventies. Now his name is not at all like his birth name. I think it must have been a way of gaining his own identity and recognizing himself as his own person.

The change was completed when he was living in Hawaii.

Today we went to the Recorder's Office at the county seat to see about copying his name-change papers. The lady there said they couldn't help. She could not explain clearly enough so I could understand why she couldn't just copy the papers and keep them on file. She kept saying only that she couldn't. So I called Hawaii about getting copies made.

We also stopped at the grocery. Troy waited in the car both there and at the Recorder's Office. He said he preferred not to go in. I actually think he felt too weak to walk but didn't want to say it.

Troy's sister, Jocelyn, is flying in from California and arriving later today. She'll be leaving Tuesday. David will pick her up at the airport since she'll be getting in just about the time that he gets off work. She and Troy can have a chance for a nice visit as a regular brother and sister even though he is so sick. Sunday when David and I go to do the laundry, they'll have some private time to talk without us being around.

Chapter 16

I called the EMT school about getting into the class since I haven't gotten a letter yet. It was supposed to have been sent this week.

I hope if I get in I can act better than when we had CPR class in police school. Instead of going first and then standing around ignoring what else was going on, I sat and watched and listened to the students ahead of me.

One of the first things someone is supposed to ask when helping an injured or unconscious person is "Are you okay? Are you okay?" That is to see if the person can give you a response.

Listening to the other students repeat and repeat the question over and over, I began to remember when Troy was hit by the truck when he was twelve. He and his sisters and I were crossing the street on the way home from the public swimming pool. He had started to cross the street when I looked up and saw a truck running the red light. Teresa was in the street, but he had almost gotten to the other curb. Through habit I yelled both their names to come back. Teresa got up on the curb, and Troy turned around and ran back and was hit.

By the time it was my turn to go to the dummy, I had begun to cry and could barely get through the CPR sequence, though I did make it. That can't happen in this class! How can I expect to pass CPR if I'm hysterical?

The lady I spoke to for EMT school said that she didn't have the information yet but would call me Monday.

Saturday November 21

Jocelyn and Troy seem to be having a good visit. This is probably the first time that they have been able to get together as two adults. It is also the first time when Jocelyn hasn't had to be mommy to her own kids for awhile. Fortunately, she was able to leave them at home with her husband so she could come by herself.

Jocelyn's adventure in the country begins. She told me there was a cow in the yard. I didn't look and told her it was a horse since the neighbor's horses get out and come over a lot. She insisted it was a cow! There might not be a lot of cows in the city, she said, but she knew what a cow looks like! When I finally did get up to look, it *was* a cow!!! It was lying down. I took a picture of it. It was neat having a cow in the yard, even if it belonged to the neighbors, or maybe *especially* because it belonged to the neighbors. It is nice having big animals nearby and not having to take care of them. I guess that is part of the reason we moved here to the country: being near the animals. We really didn't expect to have a cow lying in *our* yard, though.

I'm getting a rash on my right wrist. Peculiar. Maybe it's just a reaction to the rubber gloves. I use them all the time and to wipe off the toilet seat after Troy uses it.

Jocelyn and I put the armoire together we bought for Troy's clothes. Now the room looks pretty nice. He doesn't seem to be really concerned with it, though. He is feeling tired all the time. But at least he's getting peace, I think, and that is more important than how the armoire looks.

Sunday November 22

David and I did the laundry while Jocelyn stayed with Troy. They both just laid around, slept, talked, and "vegged-out" while David and I were gone. And worried about how to keep the woodstove going.

Then she and I drove around, and I showed her some of the nearby small towns that I like, the countryside, and some of the dirt roads.

We had pizza for lunch. David and Jocelyn had black olives only on theirs, and Troy and I had black and green ones.

Monday November 23

Our friends bought the wheelchair for Troy. That was really nice. They also got to meet Jocelyn.

Maybe I can take Troy to the hobby store and he can get something to do while he's lying down so he can keep his mind occupied.

A lady and a doctor from the Health Department visited this afternoon. She said I need to apply for Medi-whatever for Troy. I'll do that tomorrow morning, and Troy and Jocelyn can have some more time together before Jocelyn leaves.

The lady from the EMT school called and said I'm *not* in the class. I'm thirteen on the waiting list! I'm aggravated and disappointed, but I'm also thinking again about nursing school.

Chapter 17

Tuesday November 24

I went to Family Services this morning. I've got so much information about agencies I don't remember which does what. I guess I'll have to make a chart. I still haven't sent Troy's information to Social Security since I had to take it to Family Services first.

I took Jocelyn to the airport this afternoon. Troy stayed home. He said he thought he would be okay. He'll lie around. Jocelyn and I shared Nachos Grande Taco Bell and had a short farewell chat together.

Wednesday November 25

4:51 PM

Snow today? Maybe, but it seems doubtful. I got the paperwork for Medi-whichever and Social Security done enough to send in to be looked at. I need to be told what needs to be finished. I also washed a *big* bunch of dishes. Life goes on.

Troy and I went to the shed. When I was taking things out and putting them in the back of the truck, I looked at him through the back window and thought how we used to do things together. Now he is only able to just sit and wait for me to do whatever it is I have to do when we go someplace. In a way, I am accepting there are things he can't do anymore. It is an acceptance in only a minor *intellectual* manner. I can't accept it in a "total feeling" manner.

Then we went to the Chinese restaurant next to the Laundromat where David and I go. I bought carryout and we ate in the car. After lunch I went to the grocery while Troy stayed in the car. It is so sad. He used to really like to go to grocery stores, but he is so now tired he didn't want to go in even in the wheelchair. One time he told me that he was sorry that he didn't eat more deli food. He was always trying to eat healthy food and take care of himself even after he found out he was HIV positive.

We stopped at the post office on the way home. I mailed four résumés and will mail another on Friday.

Other than that we didn't do anything else.

Three years ago this morning I started to work at State University.

Chapter 18

Thursday November 26 (Thanksgiving this year)

No snow yet. According to the Weather Channel it's pretty much blown northeast or east. Troy hasn't eaten much at all. I offered him things, but he didn't have an appetite. He says it still burns when he has a bowel movement, and he's ready to die. I'm still denying and won't believe it, of course.

I remember that for so many years I used to tell Troy and his sisters that I wanted to put them in a paper bag and keep them in the living room where they'd be safe. That way, every so often, I could look in and say, "Are you all right in there?"

I wish that were possible. Sometimes I don't care how sick Troy is; I want him to stay here forever.

Chapter 19

Friday November 27

The visiting nurse examined Troy's lesion today, and it seems to be draining more.

He is still easy to care for, though. I wipe off the top and bottom of the toilet seat, the handles, and the rim of the toilet bowl with a mixture of water and bleach that I keep in a bucket behind the toilet. We use disposable pants that I line with a soft paper towel and change as needed. I use about a package of paper towels for myself about every day and a half since I've gotten tired of wiping my hands on my personal towel all the time. It gets really wet from all the hand washing I do.

Chapter 20

I called the nursing school and found out I won't be going there either. Most of my credits are so old that they won't transfer, so I would need to go back to college. *That* would take about two years, and *then* there would be nursing school, which would take another two years. I'd be almost sixty and just don't think I'd like to start over then.

Afternoon …

Troy is in the hospital again!!! We went to see the doctor, and he said that Troy should go into the hospital for a while or he'll get worse. Troy started to cry when the doctor left and we were hugging. Unfortunately, we were interrupted by the nurse with a call from the pharmacy that we'll start using. Troy was really frustrated when I got back to the room after the phone call. He said he really could have cried, and he needed to, but we were stopped.

I keep feeling so sorry for him. He's helpless in many ways. I don't care what kind of disease he has, he is still my son, and I love the person I know.

I respect him since he worked every day until he went into the hospital in Chicago. He worked evenings and sat outside in the cold waiting for a bus so he could ride to his stop and then walk home.

When he was stopped on the street and asked for money, he would take the person to a restaurant and buy them a meal. His friends that

I met in Chicago were nice and seemed to think well of him too. They weren't all gay, although I don't know why that should be important or mean anything.

He is in a private room again, so I can stay with him. Thank goodness! Am I an over-protective mother? I don't know, and I just don't really care.

His temperature was 101.4 and his blood pressure was 80/40 when he was at the doctor's office.

Tuesday December 1: b/p 100/58 at 4:35 pm

One of the problems with AIDS is a type of blindness. We were lying in our beds and Troy was looking out the window. He said, "See all those black spots out there?" Me, trying to sound calm but actually freaking out, said "Where?!" "Outside," he said. I put on my glasses, and I finally saw! He's right. It's birds, not blindness. I gave him his glasses so he could see them, too.

"They're all going to Los Angeles," he said. "Since we're west of the Mississippi, they aren't going to Florida."

He told me later in the day that he told "Spirit" that he consciously wants to participate in dying.

His temperature has been 101+ and his blood pressure is up to 100/50–60. The doctor has suggested a bone marrow test for tomorrow to determine any additional problems at this time. He is concerned and afraid but hopes that maybe this will help decide what medication will be best to use. I have to admit, though I didn't tell Troy since this is his decision, that if it were me I don't think I'd have the test. I don't know what could be found other than AIDS. He wants me to stay with him during the test, and if it's allowed, I will.

Wednesday December 2: b/p 86/40 at 3:07 pm

The bone marrow test was done about 1:45 PM. Troy was just finishing lunch after having waited all morning. He hadn't eaten much, though I think he would have eaten more if he hadn't been interrupted.

He cried as they were beginning. We held hands tightly, and I teared up but tried to remain calm for us both. When the test was finished, he said it hadn't been as bad as he thought it would be, but he wouldn't encourage me to donate anything to him like I'd thought about at one time.

He said he could feel the marrow being taken out.

He had said earlier, "All I can think of is a syringe *t-h-i-s l-o-n-g*, and it goes through both legs at the same time, and I'm a shish kabob!"

His temperature averaged in the 99–100 range and his blood pressure from 86/40 a couple hours after the aspiration to 100/60 at 8:15 PM.

Thursday December 3: b/p 100/50 at 7:35 PM

I went into town to get my driver's license since I couldn't go in yesterday. I thought the office would be really busy, but it wasn't. I just walked in, filled out what was needed, took my vision test, paid, and was out. Then I got my hair cut on the way back to the hospital.

Troy and I have talked it over and have decided that I should sometimes use the direct conversation we have between us when I'm writing this. That way I can write what he actually says about what is happening to him.

Troy: There's a constant flow of nurses during the night like a party. Last night I didn't see anybody. Is it because I'm not popular anymore?

He eats Lifesavers continually, and I worry about his teeth since the doctor says he has a mild case of gingivitis. He doesn't brush, and I hate to nag. Besides that, I forget to remind him.

There is a commercial on TV about winning bunches of money by calling a certain number. Troy says, "Can you say gullible?!"

The doctor is concerned about Troy's weight and says if he gets down to eighty pounds he'll need tube feeding. Troy is not interested.

Friday December 4: b/p 80/40 at 7:45 AM

The doctor mentions Troy's Chicago x-rays and that what they show seems to be signs of pneumocystis. (Or Kaposi's? I wonder. He doesn't mention that possibility.)

The bone marrow didn't show anything because of all the antibiotics in Troy's system. Troy says, sounding depressed, that he doesn't think that the bronchoscopy the doctor mentioned would be worthwhile. There are side effects, possibly a collapsed lung.

Well, the bone marrow test was a waste of time! But at least the doctor tried to see how he could help Troy feel better.

Troy: I'm not afraid to die, but I guess I need to admit that I *am* going to. When I think of what's going to happen, my body begins to tingle.

I could have really cried the other day in the doctor's office. It would have felt so good! But that lady came in and said the pharmacy was on the phone.

No more machines like that oxygen number thing in Chicago! I don't want machines!!

I didn't realize all the complications that could come from a bronchoscopy and don't want it anyway. I trust you to see I'm not put on any machines or that I have any more invasive procedures. The bone marrow didn't show anything, and if a bronchoscopy did, what would it prove?! I've got AIDS and I'm going to die anyway. What is this??? I am "giving up"? "Fighting to stay alive more comfortably"?

Me: (trying to be encouraging): Perhaps we need to think about *quality* of life rather than *quantity*? (How simplistic that must sound to another person, someone who wants to live more than anything else, perhaps afraid of what's ahead of them after dying?)

Saturday December 5: b/p 104/60 at 8:15 AM; Blood oxygen 98 percent lying down

There is a bald person down the hall from Troy's room, and I watch the person and a visitor together. The nurse is feeding the patient, and I think how it seems that we go from babies who can't talk to adults who can't talk. The beginning and end of our lives seem to revolve around urination, bowel movements, and being fed. This is not an unusual thought for someone in the hospital, but it's something I've never thought of before.

Troy says he thinks he'll die next year. He says he can see '93 but he can't see '94. He frequently thanks me and says I do so much. Maybe I do? There *are* some complicated things, so I appreciate the fact that he says it. I am really grateful for having the chance to take care of him now.

"Just think," he says, "you'll have fond memories of me sitting on a bedpan!"

Sunday December 6: 6/p 96/58 at 6:45 AM; 100/60 at 9:10 PM

Troy's doctor's associate came in today, and we had some laughs. He didn't know who I was just sitting there in Troy's room, so I introduced myself. I said I probably looked like some woman wandering through the halls asking if I could change dressings. He laughed and seemed to think that sounded pretty funny.

Monday December 7: 6/p 90/50 at 9:30 AM; 80/46 at 3:35 PM

We're both ready to go home, but Troy's temperature has been over 101. He's still not *really* eating, though he had half a cheeseburger, pickles, and onion and a bite of pie. He had said earlier that he was hungry and really wanted something to eat. When he began to eat, he said he could finally taste food again! We asked what he wanted most and he said a cheeseburger. I'll get him anything he wants to eat if he can enjoy it again!

He's had only one bowel movement, at 7:15 AM, but hasn't urinated. Mucus is in his throat, and his mouth is dry. The top of the insides of his mouth is very enlarged and light purple. Kaposi's? I wonder about telling him and then wonder *why*?! What good will it do for him to know? The doctor looks in Troy's mouth when he visits, so *he* knows.

Troy had an Imodium and a muscle relaxant and slept all night except for nightly pills about 3:30 AM. It was much better than Saturday night to Sunday morning when he slept only from about 1:00–3:15 AM either because of bowel movements or vitals. The nurse put a sign on his door during the night: "Give medicine *only*!"

I think Troy's really starting to "actively" die. His doctor said he'd have Hospice contact us. That's something he'd discouraged when we first saw him.

After the doctor's visit earlier, I went outside Troy's room and asked the doctor if Troy is really dying, and he said yes. He'll tell the nurses to let Troy sleep through the night. He slept most of the day and talked only a little.

When we get home I'll find out how I can get Troy the massage he's been wanting lately.

Tuesday December 8: b/p 92/60 at 9:00 AM

Troy says his mouth feels "bloated" and he's not tasting well again. He is better today, though, than yesterday.

A lady from Hospice came in. They offer a lot more services than the regular Visiting Nurses.

Troy's chart says to prepare for discharge Thursday, but his doctor says that since the weather prediction for tomorrow and the next few days is supposed to be sleet he could go home today. By that time, though, it was 4:00 PM and we decided Troy should relax and go home tomorrow morning.

5:30 PM

Now I'm worried and have mixed feelings about going home. It'll be nice going back to our little "mole hole", but then *my* responsibility begins. I'll need to figure out again what to cook, and I won't be waited on any longer by being able to go down to the cafeteria for meals whenever I want to. It makes it very easy to see how prisoners can become institutionalized.

Watching an ambulance leave, I think how reassuring sirens have been to me: "There's someone coming!" Years ago, when Troy was hit by a truck, I kept listening for the siren so I could know that someone was on the way to help him.

I called the EMT school again. The lady there said that the only thing that will help place me higher on the waiting list is to affiliate with a department. Since that's not possible, I guess I won't get in the class after all.

Chapter 21

Wednesday December 9: b/p 88/56 at 9:00 AM

Troy was discharged today, but it took *"forever"*. We thought we could just leave in the morning, but by the time the doctor got here and got the discharge papers ready and we left the parking lot, it was 3:00 PM. I had left the truck there when Troy was admitted so that whenever he was able to leave, it would be there and David wouldn't have to leave work to come and pick us up.

The doctor doesn't think Troy has long to live. As Troy was leaving the room, the doctor turned to me and said softly, "If he bombs, let me know."

Troy: About AZT. Let's not buy it. It's supposed to be expensive.

Me: Well, it's supposed to help you feel better.

Troy: It's just to prolong the onset of the disease.

Me: If it helps you feel better, I think you should take it, but it's up to you. I know I come across pushy, but it's still your decision.

Troy: We'll see when we pay for the next batch of meds.

9:30 PM

After we got home and I had put everything away, I cleaned out the refrigerator, counted out Troy's pills, changed his dressing, and sat down to share some clam chowder with David. It was about 8:00 PM.

Now it's hard to believe that we've been in the hospital, and Troy is still sick even though he's sleeping in his bedroom.

I was really stupid and didn't think about having him walk at the hospital, so now his legs are weaker. He barely ate anything while he was there, so that is making him weak too. He hasn't wanted anything to eat since we've gotten home, although he did say he'd drink an Ensure. He *did* walk to the bathroom. He'll go in there instead of using a bedpan now that he can get out of bed. No worry about that for awhile, though, if he doesn't eat!

Thursday December 10: b/p 100/38 about 11:30 AM

Our first morning home and we argue; though I don't like to think of it that way, of course.

Troy can't decide if he needs to get up and go into the bathroom or not. I've been trying to encourage him to go in if he thinks it will make him feel better. I will help him walk in there or get a wheelchair so he can ride.

Then he farts.

Troy: Well, it's gas. I guess I don't have to have a bowel movement.

Me: No wonder! You haven't eaten in four or five days. Two weeks.

Troy: Why do you say that, Mother?! I had breakfast at the hospital yesterday. And food other days. I *can't* eat a lot! It makes me sick. I'm going to stop eating eventually and die. It's as simple as that!

Me: I'm sorry. Sometimes it's just difficult.

Troy: It's something we'll just deal with.

Later, his stomach growls. He's asleep.

Saturday December 12: b/p 88/50 at nurse's visit

I put up the Christmas Tree. It's plastic. The lowest shelf I have is still too high for the ceiling, and I've had to leave the top off. It's ugly and silly looking, but there's no middle section that I can take out to make it shorter and look better. I haven't put lights on, though I may. There will be only decorations. I did put lights around the top of the kitchen cabinets at the ceiling. They look nice and rather festive. I wish the tree looked better.

Monday December 14

It's weird to be up at 11:00 PM and not wonder what the guys are doing at State University, though obviously I *am* wondering about it. I wonder if they'll invite me to the shift Christmas party. Will no one call? Or if they do will they be afraid to leave a message? One of the other officers was invited back last year after he'd been gone nine or ten months. That officer was a guy, though. Maybe they won't call just because I'm female. How will I know the reason, though? Maybe they just aren't interested in my being there; or maybe they won't even think about asking me. Men are really stupid about things like that: like I'll take it "wrong" if they ask me to the party but I won't understand that it's not really personal but that that they've invited me just because we used to work together. It's not like at the Canyon where a friend was a friend was a friend, no matter what, male or female!

Tuesday December 15

It's 3:00 PM, and it's starting to snow. The snowflakes are so pretty. They are like the flakes in snow globes, big and easy to see, falling straight down. If we were to go outside it would be quiet, the air still and fresh. Maybe the snow will stick. Troy and I both hope for snow.

Teresa sent me a really nice travel diary of her trip to Washington. It has pictures she took and her own narrative. I'd really like to go with her again.

Wednesday December 16

Troy voluntarily drank some Ensure. It's practically a "first"!

I'm getting *big* lines under my eyes. Maybe turning the overhead light on when I help Troy into the bathroom at night makes me squint. I'll ask him if he can see well enough by the nightlight.

I heard a cardinal calling outside Troy's window this morning. It said, "Birdy, birdy, birdy."

Troy went with me to Job Services. It wasn't cold, so he waited in the car and rested and slept. It took only about fifty minutes to go there and back. Certainly better than the four hours it took in Chicago! Since Chicago is so big, there are many more people to process. I still like Chicago, though.

I was told that my unemployment benefits will run out in February, and I'll have to have my case reexamined. I'm not going to tell David about all that until it happens though. He's got enough to worry about.

I also stopped at the EMT office and was told that I won't get into the class at all even with all the people who have dropped out already. There was an exceptionally large number of people who already belong to emergency departments and *have to* attend class so that they can be certified.

When I'm depressed, all I can think about is all the bad things and "no's" that have happened this year, since June, actually, beginning with Mother's accident. She and my dad still won't move here.

David's parents won't move here from northern Ohio either.

We will have to go to whoever gets sick, and so, selfishly, I would like them to be here in town where it would be so much easier to help them all.

Because I take up my time thinking about all those negative things, I forget the special time that Troy and I are sharing now, able to talk to each other as adults with adult ideas and philosophy and outlooks.

Thursday December 17

Since Troy has been concerned about his teeth, I was able to find a dentist who would clean them for him. So we got there and *waited*!!!

After about fifteen minutes past our appointment time, I asked the receptionist when we were getting in. Troy was weak and uncomfortable sitting in the wheelchair. It turns out that the dentist is an oral surgeon and doesn't *clean* teeth. I'd asked about that when I called and had told the lady that Troy has AIDS, so it wasn't like they didn't know! So I came home and called a friend who recommended someone else. Troy now has an appointment in January.

Friday December 18: b/p 90/60 at 9:45 AM

I wonder if Troy feels that he will die soon even though he says he feels he has another hospital stay coming. We are watching *The Sound of Music*. He says he'll be dozing off, and I shouldn't worry. So I watch the movie and think I must be getting old. Maria is singing about adventures, and I can't believe I'll be having any more. Having adventures seems all in the past.

I'm also getting depressed with all the *sunshine*!! That happened at the Canyon, too. I'd like a little clouds and grayness for variety. I hate all-sunny days, day after day! There are about five-plus inches of snow in Flagstaff according to The Weather Channel, so there's probably snow at the Canyon, too. Am I missing the Canyon because of the easy days there, even though I always felt that it was a "resting period" in my life?

Troy is awake now, and we start singing the movie's songs.

Troy: Dances of that time were so elegant.
Me: Yes. I think we've given up a large amount of elegance in life for freedom of expression.

We're running out of newspaper to burn in the woodstove. I'll have to ask David to start bringing home the newspaper every day. He'll also have to order more wood. Building fires is so different from just flipping a switch when the temperature goes down. I still haven't learned to build a good fire yet. David has to start one for me. Someday we'll get a furnace.

I wash my hands all the time, it seems—sometimes four or five times in ten to fifteen minutes. I want Troy to live as long and as comfortably as he can, so I need to make sure he doesn't get some kind of errant germ.

I worry about what will happen if I don't get a job and my unemployment runs out. How will we pay the bills? That is so silly since I keep forgetting that David is working.

I've applied to at least a hundred places for a job. So many ads were for companies with post office box addresses only, no company name. I can't tell if I sent duplicate résumés to the same place.

The economy is bad. The unemployment office is full when I go in.

I think companies read my résumé or applications and see when I started working and think I'm too old to work since I'm not in my 20s or 30s any longer. Or maybe it's the fact that I mention on my application that I was a security guard at my last job, and they imagine a big, brawny woman who muscles her way in to work and orders the customers around.

And then there's the fact that I'm not "bubbly". I *can't stand* "bubbly"! There's also the phony voice that receptionists use sometimes. They are just "so cute"! Yeck! Maybe I am just not right for the business world even though a receptionist at the doctor's office said I seem like "a nice enough person" when I told her I'm having a problem finding a job.

My feelings go from questions about what will happen when Troy's dead to general depression (which I'm beginning to think is a normal state of mind for me lately). But why shouldn't I be depressed because he's dying?

In the movie, Maria is saying that Reverend Mother says that when God closes a door he opens a window. Oh, really???

Troy is so appallingly thin. Touching his wrist is like touching a piece of wood. It doesn't feel soft like mine does. Vocally and mentally he is the same, though, and I can't believe that someday he won't be here.

I am planning on having him cremated and buried in the front yard either under the big tree that's beside the water pipe or by the weeping willow tree in the front part of the yard east of the house. I think about when he's not going to be here anymore and then almost immediately deny that he won't. I can't believe that I think about *burying* him. Just the thought practically takes my breath away.

The Board of Regents at the university decided today that the police substation will remain open on campus at least until June. That probably means there won't be any more university security officers being rehired.

Saturday December 19

There was a watery-looking blood stain this morning on the paper towel I use to line Troy's pants. I'm not going to tell him. What good would it do? He can't do anything about it, and it may scare him more than he is now.

Troy: I think of all the things I used to do and took for granted, and how, now, I need to *plan* before doing something. And I think about the people who haven't ever been able to do certain things, like blind people and deaf people. I realize how *they*'ve never had the opportunity to take things for granted. I still try to do things like I used to, like hurry when I walk. I'm also looking forward to spring and summer when I don't have to seek warmth under a blanket.

Sunday December 20

David and I went to the store today for groceries. He bought a Fry Baby so I could make the corn fritters Troy's been asking for. I haven't made them for years. They're light and not like the lead lumps they sound like.

Troy: I'm beginning to realize how much I have to take it easy. Like now, if I don't rest a while before I get completely up, I'd pass out if it weren't for the walker or you to hang onto. It's difficult to *realize* the situation. It's not the *experience*; it's what you do with it.

On the way home from the store I told David that I'd really like to buy the farm down the road someday. I'd also like *big* horses—Clydesdales or Belgians. But it's just a dream that actually I don't really want even though sometimes I think it would be nice.

I guess it's because the place reminds me of where I did most of my growing up.

I could walk outside to the barns if we lived there now and be a child again in my mind. But it's just more earthly ties.

I had a very nice childhood. I was really fortunate having parents and a grandmother who loved me and practically spoiled me. They could say no, though, when necessary.

Maybe it's a spiritual thing? If there's reincarnation, I *don't* want to come back again as a child. It's not that I had an awful childhood at all. I just don't want *another* childhood. That is so silly, though. How else could I learn to become an adult?

Maybe it's just time for me to move on spiritually. When Troy dies, if there's nothing else going on, like Mom or Dad being sick, I would really like to go to the Zen Center in San Francisco and get away for awhile, I think. Or maybe it's just that I want to escape?

Monday December 21: b/p 90/60 at 11:00 AM

Troy: I figure each time something new happens I could worry and get bent out of shape, but it seems best just to let it go. I don't know if there are purple spots (Kaposi's) on my lungs. Do I *want* to know?

This may sound stupid, but I want to know if I'm going to die soon. I know I will, but it's the only thing in my life that's unpredictable. I did all my moving to other cities and did it well.

The moves all went really smoothly. Spirit was really helpful. Sometimes, He helped me to find apartments, even before I got there. People I knew would tell me about places to look at or people they knew who could help me. It also happened that way with jobs. I didn't always have a job. I'd just move and find one I liked.

But this move is *death*. All I can do is go with the flow. Relax. Don't struggle. That's not good. It'll happen. The detachment is from the world. I'll step out of this body and be on the other side. It'll be a spiritual treat, I think, moving that way. There's all that spiritual ... I don't have the word for it. I'll be able to grow and continue to study, continue to move on to the higher planes. So someday it'll happen.

The only problem I'm having now is that I don't know *when* it will happen. Where will I be? Will it be in the truck on the way to your job interview? At Taco Bell? At night? Slip away. In the morning, it'll be, "Surprise! Troy's dead!"

I think it's closer. It was nice that Jocelyn was able to come. Do you understand how I feel about doing all this stuff?

Me: Like you're curious? What else? If that's all, that's okay.

Troy: I know I love the people I've been in contact with. There are people I don't appreciate, but they're outside the circle of "family" and don't count. All I can do now is ask myself what's next. I'm so weak now. At night, I go to the bedroom. In the morning, I go to the living room. If there's nothing to do I just lie there and watch TV. Then I go someplace and I bitch and moan.

Me: I don't think you do that much. I think you're letting out frustration. You've always been so active and have done so many things. It must be very frustrating now to need to plan so much ahead and not be able to do anything without having to think about it first.

Troy: If I were to say I'm scared of something, it's losing more weight. But what can I do since I'm not hungry? I know the body "eats itself," and something has happened in my left hip and femur. I don't want to get dependent on other people and ask you to do this and that like my slave.

Even if I use the wheelchair, how can I get out to the living room if I'm too weak?

Tuesday December 22

Troy used the bedpan for the first time today rather than go into the bathroom. He'd been using the urinal regularly before, ever since we got here from Chicago so he wouldn't have to get out of bed if he was in the bedroom. I've lined the bedpan with toilet paper, and, unless he has diarrhea, which he hasn't had for quite a while, it should be very easy to clean and dump out. I use rubber gloves, of course, and after I empty it, all I have to do is wipe it out with bleach and water.

I wish we could get G.O., our youngest cat, a kitten for him to play with, but L'Orange, our oldest kitty, wouldn't be able to handle it. So I played with G.O. today, chasing him around the house until he ran into my ankle and seemed to hurt his head or part of his body. He made little mews and hid under the bed for awhile. Poor little boy. I cuddled him twice. Finally he felt better, and now he's okay.

2:30 PM

Troy said he wants to use the wheelchair to go out into the living room. Is it because he's starting to use the bedpan in his room and the wheelchair will help him get around more easily and he will "feel" more mobile even though it will mean he won't be walking?

There are times when I feel an attachment to earthly things, while *he's* withdrawing. I want to feel more spiritual instead of feeling attached. I guess it's an affirmation for myself that "Hey, *I'm* alive!" There's a certain feeling of guilt attached with that too.

Troy: It's a team effort to make it easier *on* you and *for* me.

Children are the parents' karma. All the things parents need to know are learned through interacting. With moving, you know where you're going. With most diseases you know what's going to happen. With AIDS, it could be anything. You can't let it freeze you into inaction. You need to be in control.

Will I have a heart attack? What happens when I get to eighty pounds? I'm coughing and I'm so tired. Why can't I just *die*?! I'm just so *tired*! I could say it's fun when I look at it from the perspective of eternity. It's just a dot.

I'm really lucky I'm not in pain. A friend of mine was taking morphine since he was in so much pain. He was purple from Kaposi's. I mean *all over* his body, even his face! And those places *hurt*! I hit one of mine the other day. I'd rather just be uncomfortable; not take pills or feel drugged. I know my body's eating itself. I can feel it. It's like being in limbo, to not know which way is up, which way's down, which way's right, which way's left. It's like being in a void.

I really *do* love you, but sometimes when I say it, I'm reaching out to stabilize myself. My world's spinning, and I'm trying to open myself up. People said I'm brave, but I'm not worried about *death*, just the steps leading up to it. For instance, I've started coughing.

I wish I'd never learned how *not* to cry. I remember coming home from school and wanting to cry because the other kids made fun of me saying I looked ugly. And now, when I look at pictures of myself then, I see a nice-looking little boy. I was handsome.

When I tried crying at the doctor's office, we were interrupted. I feel like I'm in a swamp trying to pull myself up and grasping at reeds. That's the picture I just saw at the moment. It's not so hard, but there are certain things my mind touches once in a while, and I'm scared. It was like a big black thing. The flipside is happiness and joy. It was like being relaxed, knowing God's there and that I'm loved. We're all loved. It gives me support. It's like the black times with blood pressure, when I'm woozy. I'd rather go through that than pain. But if the pain means freedom, then it's a purifying agent that helps to clean. Pain burns karma. It's like we're at a river and I'm doing all my dirty laundry and you're doing your dirty laundry.

Me: I think that right now some of *your* dirty laundry may be *my* dirty laundry.

Troy: Yes. I guess I'm scared, but I can't let it control my life. It's nice that there's nothing to do today. Tomorrow is the doctor. Thursday is the nurse. Friday is another "free" day. But there are still things that take up time ... medicine and things that fill up the days. I feel like an old man in ragged clothes who's asking God to take him.

Me: That's what my grandmother said the last time I saw her. She said God would visit her at night. She would ask him if it were time for her to die yet, but He said it wasn't.

Troy: I look at people walking down the street; I'm not jealous, though. Their experiences are their experiences, and I don't want them!

We can have chicken for breakfast. I need to bring my focus back here. It's Tuesday of Christmas week. I'm here. Life isn't set in stone or concrete. The possibilities are endless.

I remember at the beginning of the year; I just thought it was part of the AIDS thing. I'd be so tired I'd need to sleep and eat and rest.

I didn't know I was sick when I came here. We have so much to be thankful for: a one-floor house, the small area around the toilet where I can brace myself against the wall.

Wednesday December 23: b/p 98/70 at 10:00 AM

About 4:00 AM

Troy: Life is like an old shoe that's comfortable and you don't want to give it up. A nice summer day would be the time to go, kind of warm and pleasant. I could deal with it better if I could know a date.

Me: There's people that have been given two months but have lived two years.

Troy: There's two phases: I just don't know, and I don't want to die. (*He talks softly about machines and bodies being machines. I try to write what he says, but I keep falling asleep and finally give up. When I finally wake up enough, I hear him still talking.*) I don't *look* sick, but I *feel* sick. I don't think I *act* it. (*He does look sick, but I can't tell him that. He hasn't looked in a mirror in a long time, and I would like him to keep the good image he has of himself in his mind.*)

One thing that flashed in my mind is that it's *my* experience, and why should I feel guilty about babying myself if I don't let the sickness get in control? *I* need to remain in control. For a while, though, I wanted someone else to be in control.

I read about small animals and that they feign unconsciousness so the bigger ones don't attack them. I think we all do that at some time. I feigned "unconsciousness" for a whole year. When the doctor prescribed medicine, I didn't take it. I figured if I were going to die, why take it?

And then I started getting sick. The question comes up, what would I change? There is nothing I would change. Why would I? The reason is that all experiences have meaning and "needed" me to experience them then. If I didn't, I'd do it at a later date.

I guess I should quit asking to die. Spirit knows I want to go.

Maybe I need to surrender my attachment. I have an attachment to death. Perhaps that's weird, not having an attachment to *life*. I don't have any attachment to a person. I don't have any attachment to food unless I'm hungry.

The thing about death is that it is a birthday party. We forget that. We're looking at it from this side. The ending of a life is when a person gets out of their skin and goes to another plane. On the other side it's a different plane from here: family members who have gone on before.

2:30 PM

Me: What do you think about a feeding tube?

Troy: What do *you* think about a feeding tube?
Me: I don't want to influence you. Tell me first.

Troy: I don't think I want it. Maybe it would increase my weight but still not make me better. Now what do you think?

Me *(hesitating because I brought up this discussion so I could find out again how he felt and if he'd changed his mind)*: I don't think it would be a good idea. At least if the tube were for *me*. Perhaps it's because I'm older and not sick. I don't know what I would think if I were younger, and how much I would value life if I were terminally ill. I don't know, but it seems like a waste of time. Maybe I'd get to 100 lbs., but then I'd still have the tube, well, all my waking hours.

Your doctor said it would be twelve hours a day, but it's not removed until you cough or gag it out, so it's really twenty-four hours a day.

Would that help me drive around and see the cows and hills and trees and birds or go to the mall?

He said even if it's not attached to the feeding machine, it would still be sticking out of your nose. So is that *quality*? It sounds like a longer life with a tube out your nose to me.

Troy: I still don't want it.

5:30 PM

When Troy first got here he could not sit easily because of his lesion. Now he has difficulty sitting up or standing because his blood pressure is getting lower. At the doctor's office this morning, it was 98/70. On the way from the house to the truck as we were leaving for the doctor, he could not walk all the way and had to sit on the ground for awhile. He didn't want to use the wheelchair.

We've slept practically exhausted from the trip to the doctor from since about 3:00 PM till now. *I* have anyway. Troy is still asleep.

There was one call about 4:00 PM from the Job Service about a part-time job. Then David called about 4:30 PM about needing groceries.

Then I tried meditating. Troy and I have talked about meditating before, and I think it's about time we start doing it again and not just talking about it. It's an excellent time to put all those spiritual questions and inclinations into practice.

I've really wanted for quite a while to make this a real little "spiritual hub" here, now that I'm not at the Canyon anymore. If I could put the same amount of care into spiritual activities as I do into for caring for Troy, and he could put as much in as he does trying to sit up, maybe we could get something going. I honestly believe, as Troy does, that we are working through a karmic debt from sometime past. So maybe the added spiritual direction is necessary. Who knows? And what is the difference if we're each from different spiritual directions from other people? We're saying the same things. We're just using different words.

Jesus said that his house had many mansions.

Thursday December 24

About 4:00 AM

Troy: I haven't taken an active role in eating and need to take the initiative. I need to go slow with food right now because I haven't been eating regularly. AIDS patients are on a starvation diet. Their mouths get that fungus and they can't taste and a lot just starve to death.

This is a good example of when I read that people want to experience a certain state. I've focused on death for so long. I wanted to be aware of what would happen, but now I'm crying because I don't want to concentrate on it all the time.

It's like when people will ask for money. That gives them the chance to experience something. It depends on the person.

About 9:00 AM

Troy: I've been thinking about the disease and think I'd rather be *healthy* and in Chicago, freezing. This is just *too slow!*

Friday December 25 Christmas

There was enough snow on the ground this morning to show David's footprints when he dumped the ashes from the woodstove in the yard. It was really pretty outside, too. There was some ice on the trees. When the sun was coming up it looked like the limbs were covered with glass.

Me: It's too bad you can't think of all this as an adventure, like Columbus coming here or immigrants sad at leaving their families behind but going to the New World for a new and better life. Each thing happening to you is like packing and getting ready to go.

Troy: Or unpacking.

Me: Yes, getting rid of karma.

Troy: I think I focused so much before on dying, "going home" and relaxing. I am relaxing here, but I have this vision of karma gotten in past lives wrapped around me like tape and worked off in each life. It can be like taking a cup of water from the ocean: the cup is confining the water from its home, the ocean, and when you pour it back, it's in the ocean again, and knows no bounds. Consciousness is the ocean, and there's relaxation when the bonds come off.

Me: It's like *The Christmas Carol*. I think it's what Dickens was getting at.

Today is Christmas, and I had to try to figure out what you give someone who's dying at Christmas. There was no way that we could pretend that this was just another day in a long line of days trying to pretend this wasn't happening.

I put the Christmas sock that Troy got from someplace on his dinner tray. I put a tangerine and two peppermint sticks in it in remembrance of all those Christmases past. He smiled sadly and would've cried except he was too dehydrated and no tears were possible. He knew right away what I'd given him for a Christmas present.

Chapter 22

Saturday December 26

Though Troy has used the wheelchair to get to the living room, he still generally likes to walk. I guess it makes him feel more capable, though he hurries from one room to another because he feels so weak. I worry about him falling onto the woodstove and getting burned. He has continued to walk out there, though.

But today, about 4:00 PM, he seemed to pass out and fell down while walking down the hall. He looked so helpless with arms and legs jumbled and his head falling to his shoulder.

8:49 PM

Troy: I just want to get through this! It's like an SAT exam where how good you do now depends on where you are in the next life. I'm frustrated and scared, though it's not controlling my life. When I yell, it's the frustration. I'm not used to all this.

David said today that if there had been water in Valle, south of the Canyon, we would never have left Arizona. But I think it was one of those things that was "meant to be." I haven't been comfortable here at this house yet and have wondered since we've been here why we are. Now I think I know. If we had stayed at the Canyon, Troy probably would not have been able to be with us. It was about a hundred miles to Flagstaff, the doctors, and the hospital. No hospice. Troy would have to have slept in the living room in our trailer. There was no close wall by the toilet he could lean on. The trailer was colder than here, though it can get pretty cold until I get the woodstove going. No, I definitely think that being here has allowed the two of us to get this karmic thing done that we need to get through.

Sunday December 27

8:53 AM

Troy: Every time I get up it takes me five minutes to stand. My head spins and everything. I know it's my blood pressure. It's just that I don't like passing out. But I don't want to stay here in the bedroom the rest of my life either. I wonder if I'll just get sicker and sicker.

I know how terminally ill people feel. I know it burns off karma.

It's scary because I don't know what builds into what. The biggest things are my blood pressure and my lungs. I've told you about attitude and attention. I don't know what the cause of some things are.

Me: You mean spiritually?

Troy: I wonder if passing out is freedom. I hang on so much to the idea of dying. But lying here, it's not like I'm sick unless I look in the mirror. Then I see I'm sick, and I'm getting a beard because I don't shave.

The night before when I got to the bedroom door, I was pleading with Spirit about dying, "From my viewpoint, I'm ready to go whenever you want. Even though there would be sadness among my own family about my dying, I'll be so happy. I'll be happy and healthy and better. And that's the important thing: I want to be better."

Will there be more pain now in the future? Will I be stuck in this room and not be able to get out? When I first got here I never did see myself dying in the hospital. If I do, I do. Hopefully it will be here. It would be so nice to die here. It would be so comfortable here.

I know you're writing this down.

Me: It's to help me help people like me when someone they love is dying.

Troy: I don't feel Death yet. Not on the Inner.

Did I tell you about my experience in Chicago? I "saw" a door that was four storeys tall. It was a massive door and was open. It was a big opening, and there was massive light. I stood there, not knowing what to do. The light was beautiful. I didn't feel like I had a choice. I was standing there. I wasn't moving. The door started closing. Two people—I couldn't see their faces; I was too far back—closed the door. I don't know if I could've gone. I didn't feel close to Death. When I do feel like I'm dying I'll let you know.

There always two sides to everything, like I look at things going on. I look at painful and at good things. When I look back they seem insignificant. I think it's because we put so much attention on the pain and that's what makes it seem so intensive and our attention is so focused on it.

I'm not scared, though. It's not like little kids standing at the bottom of the stairs looking up into the dark and wondering about the evil upstairs.

7:00 PM

Troy: If I live beyond '93, I'll be most unhappy. I feel like I'm carrying all this weight. I'm pulling something along.

8:00 PM

David and I bought a couch early in the month so that pressure wasn't being put on Troy's hips like it was when he was lying in the papasan. On the couch he can lie down with his legs stretched out. The thing we forgot was that he might not be able to breathe as well lying down all the time.

Me: I listened to everyone ask you about your coughing and forgot to look at it as "that particular incident". I looked at it as part of the disease. When I began looking at coughing and fluid in your lungs as incidents in themselves, I began to realize that those things were from lying down, not necessarily from being sick. I think we need to do what your Chicago doctor said and look at things as incidents in themselves so we can see what's *really* happening and if there is some way we can help you feel better.

Chapter 23

Monday December 28

Last week when we went to the doctor I asked about possibly getting an oxygen machine. Not a ventilator, but one like I see that people have in the stores these days. They carry the tanks around with them and have a little cannula under their nose. Perhaps it will help Troy feel more comfortable sitting up since it's so difficult for him now otherwise. Maybe it's just his blood pressure and nothing will help him, but I'd like to try. The doctor said insurance will not pay for it unless his blood oxygen warrants it, and I didn't think about asking more questions.

When the hospice nurse came Friday I mentioned it to her, and today she brought a blood oxygen measuring machine. It turns out that Troy has only a 60-80 range depending on whether he's sitting up or lying down. Normal oxygen content is supposed to be over 90.

His blood pressure at one point when he was sitting up in the living room was only 56 over something she couldn't get. So he will now get an oxygen concentrator. Maybe it will make him a little more comfortable.

Troy *(later in the morning after the nurse leaves)*: I'm beginning to space-out more. I can't understand what happens when I move. I just can't breathe and can't control my breathing. I guess my subconsciousness takes over and struggles for air. So maybe the concentrator *will* help!

Tuesday December 29

3:39 AM

The oxygen concentrator was delivered last evening. We have moved the small papasan back into the living room from his room so if he wants to sit up straighter instead of lying on the couch he can. We've padded it more so it's softer than it was before, and we've put the camping cooler in front of him to put his feet on again. Maybe having a choice of things to sit on in the living room can help him with any fluid or congestion in his lungs. It seems that one problem stops and another is there to take its place.

We push the machine from one room to another after he settles down to where he will stay for a while. Now, in the middle of the night, he's in his room and awake.

Troy: I can see how these experiences connect little things together.

Me: I think the oxygen will help. You'll have to wait to stand up. You may be a little dizzy, but you won't just flop down like you do now and black out.

Troy: Before I left, my Chicago doctor told me to watch out for all the little things because they can be an indication something's happening.

Me: We can also mistake things like we did about your lying down. Something like that may contribute to your health.

Troy: There's so much to the AIDS disease. Not everyone dies the same way. Or at the same time. Not specifically two years or three.

Me: Some of it's body makeup.

Troy: I feel better. When I was feeling bad the other day and you mentioned that we might have to leave the house for a while, I got this feeling inside like "Oh, no! I don't want to!" So it might be good to have someone come over Wednesday when you have to go to town, and we can see how it goes. I could get around here, but I think having somebody here would be good.

Me *(very afraid since having him mention having a sitter could very well mean that his health is getting worse. This is something I am still not willing to have to face yet. Even so, I want to encourage him to be careful of his safety.)*: I think starting to have someone here while you're feeling good may make you feel more at ease. It will also give you a chance to know someone else.

Troy: Like the nurse said, in the spring if you want to get out longer, we can have someone stay more often.

Me: The only thing I might do then more frequently is to go out and sit for a few minutes by the frog pond by the road.

Troy: I sit here coughing and moving. I really like the way the bed's set up. I feel really comfortable.

Me: It's all foam, no inner spring.

Troy: I'm not talking about death too much. I feel it really brings me down.

Me: It's not necessary to talk about it till you feel like it.

Troy: I was hoping to go this year, but, it's like referring to snow and …

Me: Living in Hawaii.

Troy: Yes, because it doesn't snow there.

Me: I think you'll like the living room now. The couch is closer to the woodstove, but the papasan and the canister are still away from it, so you don't have to worry about the possibility of sparks and the oxygen.

(I write about other things besides dying so people can relate when they read this and feel more at ease and not so alone. So they'll know that there are other everyday things they can talk about with each other too.)

Troy: Everyone approaches death differently. Some people go out and exercise. Others mope about.

Me: I think there's a middle road. You carry on the best you can. I don't mean only being depressed. You just live your life.

Troy: I guess one reason I want to die is to find out what it's like, where I'll live and eat, and what I'll be doing.

Don't hesitate to wake me up when you want to talk. Like you said, I'm not psychic. But if I were, it's like you said about the experiences, I can live them as they come and learn from them.

6:30 AM

Troy: I feel like my lungs are filling up. I wonder if it's pneumonia. If I have oxygen right now, though, my lungs will be relaxed and I think I need to push it out. I'm wondering what it will be. Will pneumonia kill me? I feel like giving up. If I give up, it'll allow Spirit to come in and take over and tell me what to do.

6:40 AM

Troy: I think it's better. I just got scared. I need to say this again, "What next, Spirit?" Maybe it was just that little bit of mucus at the top of my lungs. I just get all upset and fly off the handle. I couldn't be a nurse.

Me: There's a difference between what happens to *you* and what happens to someone else.

9:45 AM

Troy: I'm going to start drinking more water.

Me: Well, go ahead. It sounds like a good idea.

Troy: I will.

Me: It's not like when someone says that it's like exercise. All you have to do is turn over and get the cup. Or ask me for it.

Troy: I'll put the cup in my lap and just sip it.

Me: Yes, pretend you're at work.

This sleeping late is really something. We've been lying around later and later each day. Pretty soon we'll be up for only an hour in the evening. First it was easy getting up at 8:00. Then it was 8:30. Then 9:00. Then 9:30. Now it's 10:00.

Troy: It's like a swamp, just tugging forward. Then getting stuck. Not knowing how to get out of the mess. I'm just so glad you're here.

Me: So am I! It's really a pain having to look for work, though. I'd rather be here all the time. If I had a job I wouldn't be here much at all. So far, though, no one has offered me a job except the part-time job I had for a while before you went into the hospital.

I sit quietly for awhile and wonder to myself if all the tiredness, stress, and lack of sleep is just me wanting to avoid the inevitable.

After this conversation we finally get up. At night, I've been sleeping on a mat on the floor at the end of Troy's bed so that if we want to, we can talk to each other and he doesn't feel shut away like he's in a sickroom. We just usually sleep or are quiet, trying to rest, though.

Using the oxygen machine is going to take some planning. It is probably certainly going to help him be more comfortable when he sits up since his blood pressure is so low. His body isn't pushing the oxygen around his system well enough on its own. But we'll have to think of an easy method of getting him from the bed to the papasan or couch and keeping him connected to the concentrator as long as possible. This is only the second time we've moved it, though, since it was only delivered last night.

After we've made it to the living room and have eaten something, I go outside. Even though it's December, I can smell the water in the air. It reminds me of California, and I think of the times I visited his sister in LA and him in San Francisco. He and I used to walk, or he and David and I would drive and then walk. Troy was always a walker if he could get someplace that way, but now …

And he was always a good cook. People would comment on the meals he would fix. He had applied at the cooking school he wanted to attend in New York state after he graduated from high school, but he was turned down. They told him he would have to have a year's experience in working in the food industry first.

What would his life have been if he had been accepted?

While admitting to myself that we need to treasure these few days, however many we have together, I still will not permit myself much time to linger over the fact that that may be all we have together: a few days.

Sometimes I can't "allow" myself to think, though. I can only react to whatever the need is at the moment.

4:30 PM

Troy: There are all these little things to consider that we never had to do before. I need to prepare to move from one place to another. Can I sit in the living room, or will I move to the bedroom? Will I need to go into the bathroom soon? Can I *wait* to go?

I think it's going to be best to have someone stay with me.

When I thought of leaving to go to the new dentist next week, my skin got all tingly and I knew I can't do it.

8:37 PM

I'm in the bathroom and at my feet is another life and death struggle. There is a multi-legged insect caught in a spider web that has appeared there. Do I take the insect out and let the spider starve or let the spider find something else to eat? What is death for one (creature) may be life for another (creature). And what appears to be death from one's viewpoint may be life to another. I try to sort these thoughts out and leave the insect to its fate and the spider to its life.

I am pleased, of course, that Troy is helped by the oxygen and I think that he's feeling more comfortable. At the same time I'm sublimating the fact that his using oxygen is an indication of his worsening as also is his requesting someone here when I'm out looking for work. I've always taken him along to sit in the truck, but now it may not be possible any longer.

Chapter 24

Since I have to go out and look for a job, I called the AIDS Project, and they found someone yesterday to come and sit with Troy. It is the fellow's first time to sit with someone. Since this is the first sitting assignment for both of them, maybe they can help each other along. The sitter has a son who has AIDS and lives in another state. Perhaps meeting Troy will help the sitter.

There's not going to be much for the sitter to do, probably, except the important thing of keeping the woodstove going. The sitter apparently has a fireplace, so he'll know what to do. Hopefully, this will be a good match.

There's nothing I can do about leaving the house. Since I'm required to look for work, I think I will start going to business buildings and inquire at about five or six places. I can leave résumés or fill out applications if they're interested. There were no jobs I qualified for in the paper this week, so going door-to-door is the only way I can find something. So why not go to a bunch of businesses in the same place?

David hasn't said anything, but I think all this must be getting to him. It can't be a happy time for him. I think I will encourage him to visit our friends northeast of here or maybe to go see his parents in northern Ohio since it's a holiday weekend. He will have time to drive back and forth and still stay wherever he goes for a couple days.

7:00 AM

Troy: Today would be such a nice day to sleep in if I didn't have all this fluid in my lungs. It's dark and nice. I didn't mean to be bitchy last night when I hollered to get in here.

Me: Well, you were afraid.

Troy: Yes. It's all that mucus in my lungs. I know that you're here, and I was thinking about that. It seems like you're dealing with your part of the situation, and I deal with the "myself part" of it by myself. You can offer suggestions.

Me: You mentioned earlier whether you're emotionally involved. I think you've been sick for so long that you might be getting used to it.

Troy: "The new state of being"? It's definitely a new experience. It's like being on a roller coaster. There's always something else that people can make deals to God about: "I can't deal with mucus in my lungs, but I can deal with 'this' better. Can I switch?" I've done it myself before. I've had a problem someplace and asked to have the problem someplace else instead. So now I have this lung stuff. I realize no one is going to take hold of me and make me all right. Maybe talking like this is like coughing up the phlegm so that I can get rid of it. The thing to do, I guess, is just rest, or try to. Did David buy lemon juice?

Me: Yes, but not lemons.

Troy: I'll mix it and drink it. I just can't drink *six* glasses of water all at once. I feel like the hospital would have a pipe to stick down my throat.

I was thinking through all this, and I think it's like going into a cave: you can see in only so far because the light from the outside is there. A couple steps more and there's less light, but you're becoming accustomed to it. Then you have to turn on the "flashlight", which in this case are the inner resources. It's like we're walking along the path making our way. Our first experiences are easy and we can handle them. Then they get harder because we've had other experiences to help strengthen us and make us stronger, so that we're able to handle the new, harder ones better.

I know I can't run away. There's no place to go. We're always *here*, but Spirit is everywhere. Christians don't seem to think about that. They think that when they die they'll go to Heaven and don't realize that *this* is Heaven too. People say they'll pray for someone. God knows what's going on.

So the most persistent problem right now is the mucus in my lungs. You know when I bitch and moan about it, you loan me your shoulders and (*coughs*) ...

Me: That's why I'm here.

Troy: I think it's kind of neat, though. I think it goes back to the idea of life after death and that karma allows cause and effect. What you do rebounds and comes back so that at some point in a life you'll receive retribution for your actions.

Maybe you and I made the agreement when it was your turn to be sick. I think that, as I die, maybe the door of understanding will open up some more.

To go back to what I was trying to say earlier: I had agreed to have the experience of the disease. I was tired of the physical life and not sure if I could get old, handling retirement. I didn't start a retirement thing and also thought it would be an easy way out if I could participate in the process of death, so I got sick. In Chicago, I had the virus and cold but couldn't identify it as part of the disease. I kept pushing it off. It was hard. I had to sleep more. I couldn't eat. It all came together in October. So I never really went through what Kubler-Ross said about denial, in my own way, denying that I was getting sicker.

I'd still be working now if I could. I was planning to wait till it was visible to other people that I was sick, but it never happened.

I need to say this: I sit here and am using your shoulder to let this all out. I'm not directing it at you, but at Spirit, the energy and all this stuff.

Me: Don't worry. I'm not accepting it.

Troy: Maybe respiratory therapists make home visits.

Me: Maybe lawyers do too. I can get a regular power-of-attorney and can just take care of paperwork for you. That way if you don't feel like writing something you don't have to.

Troy: I'm kind of talked out. That's a relief.

Me: Sometimes you just need to get it out. That's what I'm here for.

Troy: All I want to do is to go to sleep and wake up better.

Me: That's understandable.

Troy: Like you said before, it's getting used to a new state of consciousness or being.

Me: I'm reminded of looking at babies in the nursery at the hospital and how they stretch out and jump and are getting used to a new environment.

Troy: *Full of life?*

Me: In a different atmosphere, no longer *having* to be scrunched up. Sometimes they don't lie flat either. Their backs are curved up like cats if they lie on their stomach. You've never watched newborn babies, have you? When they lie on their backs, they'll be quiet with their legs close to their bodies, and then all of a sudden their arms and legs or both jerk out straight. Before they were born, they had limits. They couldn't stretch any farther. After they're born it's different and strange to them and they have to get used to it. So different states of consciousness must be like that.

Troy: And then have to eventually move in it and become one with it.

(There's a pause of a few moments, and then he continues.) They say freedom is momentary balance. Freedom is in a split second. I was lying here a moment ago and it was interesting, like being on a river. The water was so calm I could see the reflection of the trees. It was like I was experiencing momentary balance. A lot of people have that experience and try all their lives to recapture it, not realizing they have it all along.

Me: That's what meditation's for.

Troy: Momentary stillness.

9:15 AM

Me: Do you want me to pull the curtains back?

Troy: Sure.

Me: It's a nice *gray* day, finally. *(I laugh.)* That sounds like the Addams Family.
Troy: Yes, like summer; all that sun! Duh.

8:45 PM

Troy: Life is a like a jigsaw puzzle: there's all those pieces and colors to put together. It's also like Hide and Seek. Soul doesn't change through eternity. We're hiding from Soul. We can say, "Oh, we're Soul." We don't lose anything; we're just gaining awareness.

Me: If we *allow* ourselves.

Troy: Even if we don't, we're setting up the experience.

Thursday December 31

5:00 AM

Troy has been coughing.

Troy: Did I wake you?

Me: No. I've been lying here tossing and turning. I worry about you coughing and not drinking water and not urinating.

Troy: I was coughing because my lungs are dry, but we can put a humidifier on the oxygen. It'll be all right.

(A few minutes of silence, except for three or four coughs.)

Me: And you need to brush your teeth. But you have a dentist appointment next Thursday.

8:15 AM

Troy: I usually think about food, so this morning I was thinking about food again. Wherever I lived, I found places that made good sandwiches. In Flag, there was a little deli in a bank. In San Francisco: Salmugundi's. They had quiche and soup. It was kind of expensive, but worth it. In LA, Yoshinoya; Oriental fast food; rice-glazed veggies, clam chowder, sauce. Three good places. Some roach coaches made some good tacos. Chicago: a deli bar on the other side of the river by the post office. I love Reubens if they're made right, no fat. They're expensive. I only went to that place twice. I would've liked to have gone more. Ohio: steak sandwiches. But the places we used to go to are gone.

I remember the vocational college.

Me: I remember when that was a little house by the YMCA.

(I come back into the room after emptying the bedpan.)

Me: I think how providential it was that the septic tank needed emptying just when we got here. It sure didn't seem providential at the time, though! I guess Spirit knew what it was doing.

(We have gone into the living room now. Troy had to lie back down. And he was using his oxygen!)

Troy: That is so scary! I don't know what I'd do without the oxygen. It's like I'm trying to hold myself together.

Me: Coming out of the bedroom just now, do you think it was like when you used to drag yourself to work?

Troy: I like being here in the living room with you guys, but if this continues I won't be able to soon. It may not be next week or the week after, but it will be soon. I don't know if I'll be able to go out to the doctor.

Me: Don't forget that the hospice has a doctor. Maybe he can come out.

10:30 AM

Breakfast: cheeseburgers with lettuce; tomato, pickle, and onion on the side for Troy. Green olives instead of pickles for me. I feel a real pleasure that Troy is hungry, we're after *quality of life*!

As difficult as it is for me to say "after Troy dies", I think I'll try to become a nurse assistant. I've decided that I don't want the responsibility of being a nurse, and so maybe being an assistant will let me see if I'd enjoy nursing before I really commit myself. Of course, once I get a job it'd better be the right one, since I'll be losing unemployment if I quit a job just because I don't like it. And then there'd be no income for me. But I need to take the chance, so all I can do is open myself to Spirit, and have someone offer to hire me, of course!

Troy: If I could, I'd lie flat all day.

Me: Well, it's up to you, but ...

Troy: Yes, all the mucus in my lungs. I'm kind of stuck out here till evening. If I were to go in there to the bedroom then I'd have to get up to come back here. When I lay down on the floor the other day and got back into the papasan by myself it was hard enough.
Me: It's too bad it's gotten so icy today. Maybe David could go visit his parents.

J, Troy's roommate from Chicago, has called. I tell him that I think Troy's Chicago doctor was so right. We need to look at each incident as a *separate* incident. It's not that Troy's just tired because he has AIDS or that he can't breathe because he's got AIDS. AIDS may be contributing, but things are still separate. His body's wearing down and needs more oxygen. His lungs might have filled up, but partly now, it was because he's been lying flat on the couch without moving much. And then he's in bed the rest of the time. The problem seems to be that sometimes you think you've handled one thing and then you need to think of another thing or about contributing factors. Then find you've forgotten something, and on and on.
After Troy hangs up the phone ...

Troy: I feel bad asking you to do things for me all the time; like just now, having you move the cooler to rest my legs.

Me: It'd be different if you could do it and were just lazy and said, "Well, I just don't *feel* like it! Do it for me!"

Later …

Troy's been dozing in his chair, but I wake him. He's told me several times to talk to him when I feel like it, if I want to talk. I know that we need to talk when we *feel* like it, not just when it's convenient. Sometime there won't be any more opportunities.

Me: I want you to realize that when we talk, especially if you're expressing yourself about being afraid or you feel like you're "coming apart", and I get a funny look on my face or get my pen, it still means very much to me to have you say what you're saying. I'm just writing it all down to reread later and, hopefully, to have it published to share with people who aren't fortunate enough to be able to talk like this with the people that they love. I'm afraid we'll lose the spontaneity of it, though. Here you are *talking* and I'm just scribbling away.

Troy: That's how you are, and it's okay.

Me (*crying, but trying not to, and writing with one hand while holding one of his hands with my other one*): In its own way, it's kind of funny asking, "Will you repeat that please. It was very important."

Troy: It's like you're taking dictation.

Me: There are people that can't talk about things like this. They get all upset and angry. This is kind of like Moses up there in the mountains. Can you imagine: God's talking and Moses is trying to chisel real fast.

(He begins to cough a lot.)

Me: I'm sorry I woke you up, but I wanted to talk to you before David gets home.

Troy: This morning having to get up and make my way to the living room was *so* difficult. The most difficult time I've had doing that. I thought I was going to die! I don't know about tomorrow. It's not so intense now since it's afternoon.

Me: You've been sitting.

Troy: Resting.

Me: I just want you to be out here in the living room as long as possible, for yourself psychologically, not just physically.

Troy: I just thought of a skateboard, just lying down on it and coming out. The other day after coughing my lungs out and trying to get up on the papasan myself, I relaxed. I need someone around most of the time.

Me: It's good for you to admit it so you won't be here alone and have an accident.

Troy: Well, I only weigh eighty-five lbs. (He is about 6'1" tall.) My blood pressure scares me. I just can't get up out of bed and *go* anymore. That's what my mind sees in the morning: I just get out of bed and walk out here. But I realize I can't do that anymore.

Me: It takes about two hours every morning from the time we wake up to get out here. Part of it is changing the dressing, but once that heals, and we don't need to change it anymore, getting out here won't take as long. I really think it's better to be like this than the people who fight it all the time. It seems more peaceful this way. All of us will die, and this can help us advance spiritually. It's just that fighting it all the time would be more difficult than meeting it head-on.

Troy: Or sideways. Just meeting it. For me, as things go on I get more tired and it seems harder to go on. I have less energy.

Me: I think it was Dylan Thomas who said, "Do not go gently into that good night," or something like that.

Troy: I don't think that there's a reason not go to quietly if you don't want to. You have to go on your own feelings.

Me: Yes. We're all different and have different things to live through. And here I am. I just woke you up.

Troy: It's just making it through each day. But I know I can't just get up, walk around. I go to the bathroom in the *bedroom* now!

Me: It's still hard for me to believe you're sick because we talk.

Troy: It's not for me!! Sometimes as I get up there's this big heavy feeling knowing what I have to do to get started every day because I know how much effort there is to put out there.

Me: Well, I heard you talking to your sitter the other day about dying being little steps. Not just like packing your suitcase and getting out.

Troy: I think life is like God slapping me in the face and saying, "These are the things you've got to learn." The harder the slap the more meaning there is. You know this is my time to go, don't you?

Me: Yes. If I freak out and say, "Don't go," don't pay attention.

Troy: I've already said how tired I am. You know how it is to make a circle so your fingers meet. That's how big my arm is. So much has happened to my body. It's ready to go. There're some experiences I haven't had yet, though, that I need to have before I can leave.

Me: I'm sorry about waking you up just now, but you'll be on the other side doing stuff, and I'll be wishing we'd talked and that I'd told you how I feel, too.

4:30 PM (Troy is drinking Gatorade.)

Troy: My throat feels smaller. I can't swallow well. That's why I asked you for the straw.

8:40 PM

I have begun reading to Troy at night while changing his dressing.

His lesion is almost healed; but until the new skin is the same color as the old, I'll still change his dressing two or three times a day. There is a fifteen-minute "soaking wait". I feel a real need to actively help him to prepare for his death. Maybe reading to him is *my* part of us being together now.

Troy: You can talk to me and tell me how you feel.

Me: Well, sometimes I just don't have anything to say. It's kind of like you're packing for a trip and I'm sitting here watching you get your stuff together. You say, "Well, I think I'll take this shirt, or this other thing. But not this. I won't be able to use this." And sometimes I may think of something and I'll say it. Mainly I just sit and watch.

Remember when David and I were living at the Canyon, and you left Flagstaff to go back to Ohio? It was very difficult for me to handle even though I knew, of course, that you couldn't stay in Flag at that time. You didn't have a job and had to move. So I thought of you as dead. It seems really harsh, but it was the only way I could handle it, because you left. *Now*, though, all I can think of is you getting ready to go on a trip. That's the only way I can handle *this* now.

Chapter 25

One of the things that Troy has done has been to thank me many times for doing things for him. I have told him that I know he would do all these same things for me, too, if I were in *his* place and needed help. Perhaps this is one of the nicest things. But I still appreciate that he tells me thanks. I have felt I can't do enough to make him comfortable, and he's cared enough about what I do to tell me he appreciates it.

6:30 AM

Troy: Thanks for helping me with the bedpan and urinal. It really makes it easier. I couldn't do this otherwise. I can't stop telling you this. I really appreciate you helping me. Sometimes I get scared thinking what's going to happen next.

Me: Maybe we need to change the way you look at this and use different words, like, "I'm really *curious* about what will happen next." If you say "*scared* about what will happen next", then you get that negative "I wonder *what will happen next*!!!" feeling. If we read regularly and make a real effort to meditate more, maybe that will help, too.

Troy: I find I'm opening up inside. Like the other day when I felt that "wash" sort of feeling.

Me: Well, maybe reading and meditating really will help, then.

Troy: Yes, we can start today.

Me: We've already started. We did it last night, and you didn't realize it since it was so easy.

Troy: You're right. I got an idea, by the way, on how to take that (expectorant) medicine so we don't spill it. Instead of filling a *tea*spoon *completely*, we can fill a *table*spoon *partially*.

Me: Sure. We'll try it later.

Troy: Each day is something different: trying to *sit up* in bed rather than *lying down* so I won't be so tired going out into the living room or almost passing out when I get into the wheelchair. How long will I be able to continue to sit in the living room? I'm planning things.

9:00 AM

Troy: I was remembering growing up and buying cherry ice cream.

Me: There's a company in town that makes cherry ice cream. We'll see about getting some.

He's talked frequently about food. He wanted to be a chef for years, since he was about twelve. He wasn't accepted by the cooking school he applied to, though. He was told he needed more cooking experience than just cooking at home and graduating from high school before going on to cooking school. He needed to get a job working in a kitchen someplace first. Sadly, it seems that people can lose the ability to do what they've been interested in. He and my mother both cooked well but can no longer do it or do it easily. My grandmother loved reading and playing cards and bingo and putting together puzzles but was blind for about the last twenty years of her life.

Me: I've got to get up.

Troy: Yes. Someone depends on you.

Isn't it strange the old things everyone talks about? You come into the world and are taken care of. Then when it's time to go, hopefully there's someone around to take care of you again.

10:00 AM

Troy: If AZT is pushing back the inevitable, why should I take it? I'm eighty-five lbs., weaker than hell! What good would taking it be?! So I can suffer more? So I can feel sick every day? I don't think so. All I need to do is take something that pushes back diseases. Do you understand what I'm saying?

Me: It's kind of like a "medicine" medicine.

Troy: I think I sometimes make things more difficult than they really are.

Me: In what respect?

Troy: I don't know. But I don't want to stay in here in the bedroom. I want to sit out in the living room.

Me: How long does it take you to feel all right once you get out there?

Troy: About five minutes.

Me: Well, in here you'll sit thirty to forty-five minutes taking pills, eating, getting ready to move.

Troy: Let's go to the living room. I'm not taking AZT until after we go see the doctor.

5:00 PM

I cooked rather flimsy "circus waffles". They're okay but not as good as the originals.

I made only a few, though. Troy said that the heat and oil were taking the oxygen out of the air even though he was using the oxygen machine. So he lay on the floor and scooted on his back to the bedroom. (That was what he did when he was a baby and couldn't walk. He never *did* crawl before he walked; he just scooted on his back. I'm surprised he grew hair and not calluses on the back of his head.)

He wanted to scoot into the bedroom. He didn't want to use the wheelchair. Did he feel more independent doing it himself no matter how he got in there? I didn't ask, though.

Troy: I'm going to stay in here the rest of tonight. I'm so comfortable I just don't want to move. My body is so much more sensitive than it was before. The least little bit of exercise, or lack of it, and I notice it right away.

8:45 PM

Troy: I think about what it'll be like later and if there are houses and what they're like and where I'll live.

Me: Maybe those are ideas for *here* and there's no need of those things there. Maybe those are just *earthly* ideas.

Troy: Like *laws*.

Me: Yes. If we can learn those laws *now*, we should not have any problems later.

Troy: Be aware that we *are* aware. That we're open to things now and we'll be prepared for the other side. *(a short quiet period, and then)* Are you all right?

Me: Yes. Are you all right?

Troy: Yes.

Me: I can't realize, though, that I won't be able to just pick up the phone and call you whenever I want to.

Troy: Yes. It will be different for both of us.

Saturday January 2

I slept really late this morning, till about 10:30 AM, because I hadn't slept Thursday night/Friday morning and hadn't napped yesterday. Troy was very frustrated and upset and asked why he wasn't eating much anymore. Was it because he tried and *couldn't*, or because he just *didn't want to*?

Troy: I was thinking this morning about being a vegetarian. It seems like I worried so often about being healthy and people sneezing on food. One of the hardest things I can't accept is that I can't walk. I like going to the grocery and picking out stuff. Now I can eat only a little bit. Sometimes on Saturday in Chicago we'd go to the grocery and make a good salad.

I get so frustrated! I feel like I'm walking down a hall with all these doors. I think I forgot myself too much and did too much for everyone else in this life. I get so upset. I have to concentrate on sitting up and getting into the wheelchair to go out to the living room. Everything I do I have to think about and plan.

Me: Don't you think that's natural? All your life you walked so many places and did so many things, and now you can't do them. You'd walk to work at the Canyon. The building was about a mile from the trailer where we lived. When I visited you in San Francisco, we walked all over except for short rides on the cable cars. Remember that time we walked up that steep hill from the BART? I felt like I was going to stroke out, and you were just climbing along. It seems very natural to me that you'd be frustrated by not being able to do anything much now.

Troy: Dad said I'd been angry one of these days. I keep thinking about all that food that I just wouldn't eat. There were bean salads and macaroni salads at the deli in the grocery down the street, and I wouldn't eat it.

Me: Maybe you'll be fat in your next life.

Troy: Don't say that and put that on me! I don't know what will happen. I was sick for a long time, too. I'd drag myself to work. And I was so cold! And so tired!

Me: You weren't ready to quit.

I remember at the airport, when you sat slumped in the seat instead of jumping up like you used to when boarding was announced. I almost asked you to stay here rather than go back to Chicago. But I didn't. So, to excuse myself, I wonder if you'd stayed if you would have been sorry. When you got out of the hospital you were going to stay there in Chicago till the spring. Then the end of November. Then you decided you'd come here.

Troy: If the apartment hadn't been so *cold*, I probably would've stayed there.

3:00 PM

Troy: You okay?

Me: Yes. But I worry about you. You need to brush your teeth. You're not using your oxygen either, are you?

Troy: I don't want to be dependent on it.

Me: But you haven't been breathing deeply.

91

10:30 PM

Troy: Today seemed to go well. I sat out in the living room and didn't cough till I got here in bed and turned the (electric) blanket a little higher. I cough and hear crackle and pop.

Me: Now that you've taken your medicine, do your lungs feel crackle and pop?

Troy: For a while there, I was going through a sugar binge. I guess it was about going to the hospital.

Me: You ate better today, too. Some days you just don't eat anything, or, like today, you ate a lot.

Troy: Yes, my taste buds work sometimes, and sometimes not.

Sunday January 3

2:00 AM

I made a "mistake" of sorts. I turned on my scanner and listened to the guys at State University. Life there seems so strange and far away, and I can't imagine it there. I am so involved with life here that having worked there is like something I dreamed. I heard a rumor that my nine-month position was open to only the next person in line from the layoff. So the other female officer took it. I doubt if I'll ever be called back. If I *do* get called back later, though, after Troy dies, will I want to go back or try to work as a Nurse Assistant instead? I need to stop pretending.

7:00 AM

Troy: I never thought I'd be at home and sick.

Me: But you did have some warning, though.

Troy: Yes, but I never acknowledged being sick. I denied it instead. It was nice that you took care of all the details of moving.

Me: There's always something in life that slips through—the people that call and don't leave messages on the machine, the envelope I forgot to put a stamp on.

Troy: They seem to be little things. They could have been big things. Like this mucus stuff. I go to sleep and there's all this mucus in my lungs. It's "Where did *all this* come from?!" I seem to be getting *more*! I was going to ask if you could call Hospice today and find out if there's any other drug to help clear the mucus out.

Me: I called the doctor, and he said there's only that expectorant.

Troy: Maybe I'll have to sit up straighter in the papasan. Yesterday before going to sleep I had some iced tea. Everything tasted so good.

Me: Maybe your taste buds are working again. Is it hard to tell when they are or aren't?

Troy: I don't know for sure. I'll have to pay attention and think about it.

Me: I wonder why you could tell so much better in Chicago.

Troy: I don't know. I think it's the fungus. I wasn't taking Diflucan or Mycelax then.

Can we have some lime sodas after dinner? We can see if it tastes like it used to.

10:45 AM (We have just finished changing his dressing.)

Troy: I think I'd like to stay in bed today and relax.

Me: Tired from all that moving around?

Troy: No. I just think it'd be nice to stay in bed for a change and take it easy.

Me: You don't feel bad and plan to do this every day?

Troy: Mother! Why do you say that?! Every day you ask me that! When we were growing up you'd sleep on Sunday afternoons.

Me: Yes, that's true. I'd forgotten that. I'd fix dinner after church and wash the dishes and sleep on the couch while your father would watch football. You're right. Everyone is entitled to a lazy day. You haven't had one since you were in Chicago.

Troy: What time will you and David eat dinner?

Me: I don't know; 2:00 or 4:00. I'll come in and let you know.

1:47 PM

I'd gone into the living room with David and then heard noises in the bedroom.

Me: Hi. I guess you're awake. Do you want to go out to the living room?

Troy: Yes. Pretty soon. I was lying here and looking at the clock and it was 1:34. That's enough sleep on Sunday for me, I guess. I'll just sit here for awhile.

Me: I'll be back at 2:00.

2:00 PM

Troy: I guess I'm holding back a lot of frustration and anger and need to talk. It's so hard to try to sit up. Will you turn the oxygen up to 3, please? I just really appreciate you being here.

Me: Would you like me to order a bigger machine?

Troy: No. I know I won't be getting any better. This is fine right now.

Troy later goes into the living room.

We've started leaving the oxygen tubing lying in a coil at the bottom of the concentrator beside the bed and backing quickly into the living room in the wheelchair. That way, I can just keep the wheelchair facing in the same direction all the time, and I don't have to keep turning it around. Then Troy gets into the papasan and settles down while I bring the concentrator in beside him. After he stabilizes, we exchange the 50 foot tubing for the 7 foot.

Today it's taken him fifteen minutes to get into the living room. He tried to sit up, then he lay down, then he sat up again several times before getting into his wheelchair so I could wheel him out. Finally, he got into the papasan ... about forty feet from the bed. We've never timed how long this takes before now.

8:45 PM

Troy: I don't know why I've been so fixated on trying to sleep today.

Me: Maybe it's because it's Sunday and also the last day of a three-day holiday weekend.

Troy: Yeah. "Back to work" tomorrow. I'm ready to go to sleep again.

Monday January 4: b/p 90/60 at 11:06 AM

Dinner was late yesterday. Did I make David mad?

I try to balance everything so that he's not disturbed and his life can still go on as normally as possible; but sometimes it seems that just doesn't. David doesn't complain about it.

9:00 AM

Troy: I feel emotionally sad. I had the Ensure. I'm at a plateau. I'm glad I didn't cough all night. It allowed me to sleep. I feel so helpless.

Me: Maybe if you—I know it sounds trite, but maybe if you read, write to people, play games, it would help you feel better.

Troy: Yes. I'm going to start to write to people.

Me: Keep your mind occupied.

Troy: I still just can't go to the other room without thinking about it. I have to go through a process. I'm not an invalid yet, am I?

Me: *(How can I tell him yes? That would make him feel more helpless and depressed. It is so negative! Talking about dying seems, strangely enough, more positive, because we both feel he will be going on to other planes and spiritually expanding and growing. But "invalid"??? Never being able to do anything anymore that he's been used to just doing before, even if it's making the effort of just sitting up.)*

I don't know. I think you should focus on what you *can* do, not what you can't.

Noon

Troy had been talking about "fun foods" all morning: Kool-Aid, Jello, cheese tortillas, pretzels. No cereals, though. Food has always been his most favorite thing, and now he's *starving*!

The hospice nurse said she'll come back on Wednesday if we don't go to the dentist, and then she'll start seeing Troy three times a week. He's deteriorated more (she doesn't say so, but I can tell) and seems like he'll need more visits.

12:30 PM

We started so late that Troy says he thinks today will be a "chickening out" day, and he will stay in the bedroom. Once he gets to the living room, he's okay, he says, but the effort of getting from the bedroom to the living room is just too much right now. We've discussed crawling or pulling him out on a piece of paper, too, if he doesn't want to use the wheelchair.

1:15 PM

We've had some lentil soup for lunch, and Troy says he's beginning to feel better. He needs to eat more than Ensure for breakfast. He says to call today's events "Chicken Day" in our book.

Troy: I feel better. Something's happening. I'm just tired of trying to go to the living room. I eat lentil soup. Before, I didn't have any energy.

My purple spots on my back are the size of moles, and it's hard to say what's happening with those until we see the doctor about them.

I feel, too, that I need to *know* that eating is important to being able to go out there. Ensure is just not enough. We've reached an impasse. When it's warmer in the other room, maybe I could crawl. Taking the wheelchair is really an effort.

Me: It's just natural, and we need to be more aware. Things just happen.

Troy: I get really frightened about things, Mom. I just can't go to the dentist Wednesday. I'm just too weak. I don't know how I'll get to the doctor appointment either.

Me: Don't worry. Dr. G's appointment isn't until the end of the month.

Troy: I'm glad these little realizations come. I'm glad I've realized I wasn't chickening out about not going to the dentist. That I realized I was just too weak to go. Remember, *NO* ventilation machines, etc. My focus, of course, is on death, because it's the next thing that's going to happen. The only way I see myself getting out of this room is with an ambulance or a wheelchair. I *feel* like myself, but sometimes when I think about what I can't do, I'm ancient.

Me: Well, that's how we see ancient people, by what they can or can't do. I think you should just take things slowly.

Troy: Do you think I'm not?

Me: No. I'm just suggesting.

Troy: My body feels kind of shriveled, and my lungs too. At night, there are all these bony points in my body. I lie one way for a while and then have to change to the other side. I try not to put attention on it. It's getting harder to take deep breaths.

Me: When you lie on your back or on your side?

Troy: On my side.

Me: Your chest is compressed. Try to throw your upper shoulder back just a little.

Troy: I'm really glad we decided not to go to the dentist Wednesday. I just couldn't see myself walking through the bedroom door, and then outside. I was worried how I could eat enough to give me the energy to get there. There was just so much to think about. It was so frightening.

10:30 PM

Today was a day that so quietly changed so drastically from beginning to end that it's hard to believe unless I look back at the way it started. This morning, Troy had an optimistic sound in his voice and he spoke with a lilt as he talked about "fun foods" and really looked forward to having some. It was so different from this afternoon when he held my hand and said he was frightened about how he could get to the dentist and doctor. Then, in the evening, he said he was relieved that he wouldn't have to go after all. How sad. Today could have been two completely different days.

I wonder if family members of the sick are somewhat "protected" in a way? The nurse made a comment one time about being able to see changes in clients that the family is sometimes too close to see.

11:30 PM

We're in bed. I've been sleeping on a mat on the floor at the end of Troy's bed for quite a while now. I couldn't always hear him call me when I was in my bedroom when he wanted to go to the bathroom or just needed me, so I moved in here. It's nicer really, because we can talk more spontaneously and I can keep him company at night if he feels lonely and will wake me up.

Me: How do you feel now about not going to the dentist Wednesday? Are you still relieved?

Troy: Welllll, I just turned over. Let me catch my breath. Like we said, where would the energy come from?

Me: Well, you've been brushing your teeth every day now.

Chapter 26

Tuesday January 5

12:35 AM

Troy *(urgently)*: Mom! Will you come and sit with me!

I've treated my disease for years like a game, and now I realize *it's real*! I'm really getting scared now. *(He asks for a muscle relaxant.)*

(I realize that I can only hope that Death will come to Troy as a friend and gently slip its arm around Troy's shoulders to help him on his way.

I put my head in my hands and begin to cry.)

7:51 AM

Troy: I'm worried about my blood pressure. I just … I just … I don't know. What's today?

Me: Tuesday.

Troy: The 5th?

Me: Yes.

Troy: It's right now; right now. *(to himself)* Relax.

(to me) I'll need another muscle relaxant. I'm not taking tranquilizers. The muscle relaxant; I may need it in the middle of the night. It seemed

like my body didn't want food. Then I ate gumdrops and my taste buds ...

Me: *Stopped* working or *started* working?

Troy: You know, I'm getting to the part where rolling over is ... I need to find another way to get to the living room.

Me: I can still take you out in the wheelchair, or David can carry you when he's here.

Troy: I was imagining getting to the papasan, arms flying. My energy levels got me. When I sat up in bed when my sitter was here, he had to help me. I spent ten minutes trying to catch my breath. It's getting to be an effort to put my legs up to urinate. It's an effort to breathe now. I'll have to eat more today. I'll have to experiment more. I'm not chickening out.

Me: I know you're not.

Troy: I'm trying to evaluate. I'm not bitching and moaning. I feel like the body is saying, "I'm weak." I'm giving in to it. It's like a roller coaster. It never ends. This "less energy" ... Oh, it's learning to do the things I need to do more simply. Maybe I'll need a machine (oxygen concentrator) that goes to 4, but all I need now is 3. It's like an adventure. Don't you have anything to say?

Me: No. I'm just listening.

Troy: I never thought I'd feel like this. It's a weird feeling. Especially when—did I say it was a weird feeling? Especially when I have to move around. Then it's intensified. I explained to my sitter how I wanted the pillow. I thought *I'd* do it, but *no way!*

Me: It's almost time to do your dressing.

Troy: You'll have to help me tomorrow when the nurse comes. How do *you* feel about what's going on?

Me: I don't believe it.

Troy: That's how I felt. I thought that I'd work and then I'd just drop dead.

Me: I'm glad that it didn't turn out that way. If it had been suddenly it would have been terrible for me. I know that's selfish, though.

Troy: Did you call and cancel the doctor?

Me: The *dentist* was tomorrow. The *doctor* is at the end of the month.

Troy: I doubt if I'll feel different. Mom, it's so nice to rest, relax, close my eyes. Three on the machine seems more comfortable.

Me: If you want more, we can call the company to get a machine that goes higher.

Troy: I'm getting to the point of asking you to do more things.

Me: That's what I'm here for. That's what *we*'re here together for!

8:30 PM

Me: Please remember when you go, if things get busy, that I love you. I don't usually tell you, so I don't want you to forget.

Troy: Yes. I love you very much, too.

Me: Or you might slip away, too, at night, and I want you to know that I love you.

Troy: Yes, I know. *(pause)* It's my own fault for not eating when you're not here and someone else is. I just space out and want to go to sleep. Well, let's see. Let's wait till nine o'clock and get medication if you can wait till then.

Me: It's only thirteen minutes. There's no problem.

Troy: I told you that '93 is the year that I'll go. I'll be happy. But you'll be going through your stuff too. I hope you'll realize that. My mind is changing, dealing with day-to-day things. Death will happen, but I don't know when. If I keep focusing on death, all the things I do in the Physical flash by, so I'm focusing on what I need to do here.

Maybe tomorrow we can have hot chocolate.

Me: With mini-marshmallows.

Troy: You said a muscle relaxant made you sick.

Me: So I had beer instead.

Troy: Growing up; that's a good memory. Peter Pan peanut butter. We'd go down to Grandma's and Grandpa's patio. Eat and play.

Me: I just flashed on a picture of Teresa; her hair, the side of her face. I don't know if I was thinking of a picture or about how she really looked.

Chapter 27

Wednesday January 6: B/p 80/60 at 11:00 AM; temp 100+ at 11:00 AM. It would not go above 96 after that.

6:00 AM

Troy is beginning to freak out. Will it be another November episode? He had a nightmare about 4:30 AM. The areas around his eyes look darker. It reminds me too much of that last time. I suggest a muscle relaxant, hoping to avoid the fear for both of us.

Troy: Fun, fun, fun, fun, fun. Happiness. What other nice words can you think of?

Me: Cats. Flowers. Birds. Yes.

Troy: Yes. Bird twitter. Sky. Clouds. *(He takes the muscle relaxant.)* Fun. *(pause)* Relax is a good word. The last time I took one (relaxant), I couldn't finish my sentences.

Me: That's because you were falling asleep.

Troy: Would you give me a shot of 3 *(on the oxygen concentrator)*?

Me: Okay. Then I'll wash my hands and kiss David goodbye. He's leaving for work. I'll come right back.

We leave the light on while the relaxant takes effect and he sleeps.

7:30 AM

Troy: I feel safe here. I denied this (dying) before, but no longer. The other stuff is still there but on a different level.

Troy dying?! *Nooooooo!* Irrational thoughts run through my mind: How can I stop this? What can I do? I'm being selfish again. I want him to be healthy and live forever.

10:30 AM

He woke me up about 10 till 10 and doesn't want me to leave him.

Troy: You've given me a lot of physical support. You help me when I make boo-boos.
Me: What do you mean?
Troy: When I have no protein but don't want to eat.
Me: You need to eat, though, and tell people exactly what you need.
Troy: That was an awful experience earlier. I was so scared. What's the time?
Me: 10:30.
Troy: At 10:35 I'll drink Ensure. That's my goal. It's not easy. The next days, I'll need to eat.
Me: You need to ask when you get hungry. *(Yesterday I had to go to town to do errands and drop off résumés. I didn't get home till almost 5:00. He'd had pizza for breakfast, and the sitter fixed ravioli for lunch, but he didn't ask the sitter for anything later.)*
Troy (Drinking Ensure): I guess I'm learning. I'm feeling better. *(small sips)* Thanks for bringing it to me. Did you get enough rest?
Me: Yes.
Troy: I'm not going to the living room today. I'm healing from the protein (Ensure). You know … *(moving around when he's finished drinking and now talking to himself)* … Relax.
At 1:15 will you start the fire?

When I was sick in Chicago, I used to give myself goals. I'm not scared. I wasn't working with Spirit. Do you need to call anybody today?

Me: I'm going to call about the room monitor. Maybe I can find one someplace.

Troy: Can you do it Friday? My heart; have you ever been with anybody and felt so much love streaming from your heart? I feel lots of gratitude and lots of love.

Me: I return it to you. Or maybe I should say I accept it. Or should I give it back? I continue to think that's why we're together—so that I can take care of you and help you to feel comfortable.

Troy: Well, as your heart gives it back, it touches mine. A big circle. After you do the fire, will you come back in?

Me: That's why I want the room monitor, so that we can both talk to each other when I'm not in the room. I can actually buy two. We can set them beside the bed and beside the sink. That way one can be used to talk on and the other one to listen on. We won't have to pick them up that way and push buttons. We can use them when I'm in the kitchen washing dishes or fixing food. So far I haven't been able to find one. I don't know why not. Even the baby store I went to didn't have any.

Troy: Is it time to start the fire? I guess there's nothing else to tell you.

Me: Will you be here when I get back?

Troy: Yes. Here's hoping the fire in the woodstove will be easy to start.

Me: Yes. I have to build it.

Oh (*yelling to him from the living room*), David's built it already. All I need to do is light it.

(It's noon, and we're *finally* eating breakfast!)

Troy: I'm so glad the nurse is ordering pain medication for me.

Me: Well, you need to say something. You've not said anything for too many years about feeling bad.

Troy: What's in the bowl?

Me: Poached eggs, just like you have. I try not to eat them too often. You know what they say about cholesterol.

Troy: Yes. It's all crap. I'm really glad I'm getting the pain medication.

Me: Please say something when you need it.

Troy: When I woke up last night I was just dehydrated.

Me: Were you in pain?!

Troy: Yes.

Me: You need to tell me!

Troy: I guess so. One lesson at a time. The medication will be so good. Maybe in a couple months we can get a hospital bed so I don't get pushed down and can sit up more straight.

1:30 PM

Another problem: durable power-of-attorney. I *knew* about it in Chicago and have thought about it here but kept pushing the thought away. I have a *medical* power of attorney, but not the "regular" one. Now I am facing what to do with papers—insurance forms, requests for *anything*! All lawyers want the person to come to them. No wonder! We'd have a party here—lawyers, notary, witnesses. But how else can it be done? I'd thought about seeing a lawyer today. *Today*?!

I'm going to find a lawyer to see if he has any suggestions. Hopefully I'm not too late to call around. But then it'll either be okay or it won't matter by the time I find anything out.

Troy has started sleeping with the oxygen at 2 ½. That's up from 1 when he first started using it.

2:00 PM

I've moved the papasan back into the bedroom from the living room. I put it in a corner. I can always put it back out there if Troy decides to go out again. But I know in my heart that that will be an unrealized dream. I'm not ready to admit he'll never go out again. So I sit here with him. I've put it beside the bed.

The hospice nurse has finally *said* he's deteriorating.

He says no water right now; he wants to sleep. I give him ice chips or feed him liquids with a spoon. It is too much effort for him even to use the straw that I've cut down to make shorter. He cannot suck well any longer. I smile and tell him that's it's like a mama bird feeding her baby bird.

I plan to wake him at 3:00 and give him Tylenol for his hip, change his dressing, give him medicine at 3:30, and then fix lunch. We'll have beef stew if he's hungry.

I want to write and write about him, hoping in some magical way that that will keep him alive. His spirit, though, is weakening. His eyes are somewhat dilated. Natural before death? Is that why he needs his glasses? To see up close? Or will his pupils become wider and wider? He breathes quickly and shallowly. And I write on hoping to put off the inevitable.

Me *(crying while trying to wake him up)*: I need to read this to you. I wrote it down a while ago so I wouldn't forget. You asked earlier how I feel about you dying. If it were myself, alone, "going", I think I'd feel rather scared but excited at the adventure, like when I went to Arizona the first time. But since it's *you,* that's different! That excitement for *your* adventure is still there, but it's mixed with very much sadness and selfishness that I won't, like I've said, be able to call you whenever I want to. You'll be off doing things, and I won't have a telephone line far enough to reach. So I want to tell you, both, "Stay! Don't go!" and "Go. Have a good time! Enjoy yourself." I love you very much and want you here with me, but at the same time I want you to enjoy yourself "after" and have fun.

Troy: Thank you. I'm going to miss you too. Who knows what we could have done or and where we all would have moved and visited each other.

Me: Maybe we've done it all.

Troy: Right. Karma's ending.

Would you get me some more ice please?

(I bring the ice in) We've got the agreement that when *you* arrive I'll be there.

Me: I don't know if I want to come back "here," to another life. I may have to, though.

Troy: Me either. I want to explore the new life.

Me: It may be more fun.

Troy: Whatever's good for Soul.

Me: It's getting time to change the dressing.
Troy: Lucky me.

This time he's really weakened. I have been taking his blankets down and lifting his legs for a dressing change or for him to urinate. He was taking off his pants himself. This time, though, he asks me to do it.

Now, after he sleeps and first wakes up, his voice sounds drugged and thick, though it improves somewhat after he talks for a while.

I wonder; do we have much more time together?

I put the thermometer in his mouth and sit beside him listening to the oxygen machine while I'm waiting for time to pass so I can take the thermometer out of his mouth.

His temperature is 97. That's what I shook it down to before putting it in his mouth.

Me: I'll take it again when you're on your back.
Troy: No. Let's just do it later this afternoon. My mouth is too dry. What time is it? Are my dressings almost done?

After his dressing is finished, I try to take his temperature again. I'm afraid, but what difference will it make if it's not higher? It's still 97.

Troy: I spaced out.
Me: I'll take it again after a while.

Dead is such a "dead" word, I think.
I'll take his temperature later.
Will he have died by then!
By morning?
"Later" is much more active-sounding. Even now I won't give in to having him gone. Will I ever ?? I think of the people I'll need to call.

Troy: Whenever I move, don't ask me any questions. I need to put out so much effort.
Me: I'll try to remember.
Troy: Stay here a while. I guess I'm going to sleep.

Me: That's all right. Go ahead.

3:30 PM

Me: I'll give you your Tylenol now and your medication at 4:00. You can have beef stew.
Troy: No. Let's wait till 5:00, then I'll have Ensure at 8:00.
Me: That's what happened yesterday. You ate, but not enough.
Troy: I *did* eat. This morning I had eggs.
Have you been able to sleep?
Me: A little.

I fix myself a peanut butter sandwich and a Coke with a little rum in it. That will be *my* muscle relaxant, maybe.

Later:

Troy: What's AZT and DUI do?
Me: I don't know exactly what they do, but I think they help prolong the symptoms or the complications of AIDS. Do you want to start taking AZT again?
Troy: No.

4:30 PM

Is Troy talking? Dreaming?
"Am I ready to go?" I hear him say.
The last time I saw my grandmother, a few months before she died, she told me that God came to visit her, and she asked him to allow her to die, but He told her not yet.

4:45 PM

I can read the Buddhist books about dying experiences, but not the hospice books from the AIDS Project. Are the books from the Project too close and too real?

It seems that Troy has slept off and on practically all day except for the morning hours between 9:30 and noon. How many hours does he have left?

4:50 PM

I have called a friend and left a message on her machine. Her husband died last year, and I guess I should take the step and admit we will need a funeral home soon.

5:30 PM

I've offered Troy beef stew twice, but he's not hungry for that or anything else I can think of.

Troy: I don't want to stay in bed tomorrow till 10:00 even if I am tired. Does my body say I'm sleepy because I really am or because it doesn't want protein? I can't understand why I'm so sleepy.
Me: You didn't sleep last night. You had dreams.
Troy: *Not* nightmares.
Me: *Weird* dreams.
Troy: I just went along with what you asked was happening. I was dehydrated. No water. No oxygen.
I'm rubbing a sore spot. It feels good. The Tylenol worked before. Not real fast, though.
I take one little sip of Ensure, and I need to rest. I've gotta drink it *slowly*.
(silence a while) Well, I'll be glad when it's over.
Me: The Ensure?
Troy: No. The pain. At least we know what to do until we get the medicine tomorrow.
(We are using a drug company that has their medicine delivered by Federal Express. Troy doesn't want me to leave him to go to the store to get any medicine, and by the time David gets off work, the store is closed. So we will have to try Tylenol in the meantime and wait for the other medicine to be delivered.)

Me: The nurse didn't think the problem is your back, but she didn't say what she thinks it is. We'll tell your doctor.

Troy: I still don't think I'll be able to get out to see him. I'm glad you and I are still pals even with those little blowups.

(He'd gotten angry with me earlier when I was trying to straighten his bed, getting him towels to eat with, and just generally hovering. He said I was buzzing around like a bumblebee, here and there, and all over.)

Me: How can we let each other know things unless we talk about them?

Troy: Talk to me about your feelings.

Me: The best thing I can say is what I wrote down and read to you earlier. That's why I wrote it down, so I wouldn't forget. Otherwise I knew I'd be upset that I couldn't remember.

Troy: I'm glad you did. (He begins to fall asleep. The Tylenol is taking effect.)

9:15 PM

Troy's taken his evening medicine and is settling in for the night.

Me: Do you want your ice cubes now?

Troy: Mother! *Slow down*!! This is like the jack rabbit and the tortoise. I'm just dehydrated. I've thought about going to the hospital to be rehydrated, but then I think, no.

Chapter 28

Thursday January 7

The oxygen concentrator broke down about 2:45 AM and we needed to call a repair man to bring another. Until he arrived, we used a portable canister. It worked okay, but I was afraid that it would stop working, too, for some reason.

I hadn't been asleep since about 9:00 AM Wednesday. I can't sleep right away when I lie down, even at night after being up all day. I can't seem to take naps. I toss and turn.

Last night whenever I would start to doze off, Troy would call out or talk to me. He was agitated about his breathing and wanted the oxygen continually changed from 2 to 3 and back to 2. I wrapped myself in my grandmother's quilt and sat on the floor till he settled down. Then I'd lie down on my mat and he'd call out again. Since he was talking in his sleep, he would have to call "Mother" sharply so I'd know he was talking to me. At 2:30 he took a muscle relaxant and I thought I could sleep for a couple of hours, but that was when the machine broke.

David got up about 4:00 since he said he woke up about 3:30 and couldn't go back to sleep either. He had to go to work though, anyway.

Troy continued to talk and be aware, talk and dream, and ask for machine adjustments till …

9:30 AM

Troy: I don't know, Mom. I don't know what to do about my health. Do you want to sleep till 10:00, and then we'll eat?

Me: We can eat now or wait.

Troy: Let's wait a little while.

11:00 AM

Troy's becoming extremely agitated, though this time, unlike the other two times, he is aware of who he is and where he is and what's *really* going on. He has asked me to call the doctor because he cannot breathe well even with the new machine set at about 4 or 5. He cannot swallow at all. Or breathe. I tell him to relax, try to be calm, and talk to Spirit, while I am running around trying to grab everything to get together if the nurse says to call the ambulance. The only way he'll be able to get into *any* vehicle is on a gurney since he says he can't sit up.

Troy: Mother! Call the doctor's office again. I can't breathe! I'm going to die! I want to go to the hospital! I'm scared! Call the doctor again!

Me: It won't do any good. We have to wait. The nurse said she'll call us back as soon as the doctor gets off the phone and she can talk to him.

I'm rushing from room to room trying to calm him, hold his hand, flinging words at him while I'm flinging clothes and toilet articles into my bag, trying to do everything at the same time. I *know* what the doctor will tell us, though.

Me: They may be able only to put you on a ventilator. There may be nothing else that can help you.

The nurse calls. She says it's true: only a feeding tube and a ventilator remain for help. There is no medication to help him with his throat.

He stops flailing and calms down. Has he decided to die?

He drinks some Gatorade. Maybe electrolytes will help.

Me: Do you want your oxygen increased?
Troy: No. Not now. Later.

He pushes the blankets to his waist and turns off the electric blanket.

Troy: Close the bedroom door, please.

He lies quietly, mouth relaxed, eyes partially open.

Me: I love you, Troy. (*I feel so helpless.*)

He shakes his head. This has broken his concentration. He takes his regular medicine, plus a muscle relaxant and the pain medicine that arrived earlier.

1:15 PM

Troy begins to doze again. I *have* to sleep also. Sometime *soon*! I sit down on the floor beside his bed and put my head on the blankets hanging down the side of his bed.

3:30 PM

Troy: I may end up leaving tonight.

I wonder if Troy is hallucinating or dreaming. He also talks about maps and places under new management. I don't want to ask and make him wake up in case he's actually asleep.

4:30 PM

I listen to Troy breathe, and I know it won't be long. I can now imagine his spirit like a little bird learning to fly toward the sky. *My little bird will fly soon.*

8:30 PM

I *finally* think of moving the papasan to beside Troy's bed where I can hear him easily and be closer to him. "Why didn't I think of this before?!" I think ruefully. "Like he's going to wake up *now* and be glad I moved this." Probably he would have been glad yesterday. Or this morning before the call to the doctor. Not now.

Chapter 29

Friday January 8: b/p 74/54 at 10:55 AM. His temperature still will not go above 96.

7:00 AM

Troy has lived through the night. He began to "rally" sometime very late in the evening and asked for stew, even though he'd fallen asleep again by the time it was heated. His voice has changed from what it has been. It's now more deep, more husky, more "elderly". He breathes a heh-HUH, a heavy exhaling sound, though not overly loudly. I had the tape recorder on this morning to record, but the tape was in wrong and didn't record.

Troy: I love you. I'm so glad to be here.

9:42 AM

Troy: I feel that I don't know stuff that I need to know about things.
Me: Ask me.
Troy: I forget. If something changes, I need to know. Does someone live here besides you and me?

Me: *(I'm scared. He's forgetting again. I try to sound calm.)*: Just David, And the cats.

Troy: I wasn't sure if we shared the house or what.

He's drinking Ensure, more easily, in a way, than yesterday when he could tolerate only ice chips. He still doesn't think he can swallow his medicine yet, though, since they're pills.

12:25 PM

The hospice nurse has come and gone, leaving behind such a simple medication direction I'm upset I didn't think about it: crush pills and put them in a tablespoon of juice! My mother used to do that me when I was a kid. I can't believe I forgot!!! So he took some pain medication in pineapple juice followed by Gatorade. He doesn't want his other medication yet, though, he says.

What do I do as a Caregiver? I can't *force* him to take something he doesn't want, and so far he can't be *persuaded* to take it.

1:06 PM

My lunch: a beer and a peanut-butter-with-banana sandwich.

I've washed the urinals. They're practically like new; no old-urine smell. I rinsed them out, added bleach, rinsed, soaked with bleach a couple minutes, rinsed, bleached again, rinsed, two washes with my gloved hand on top to keep the water inside, more rinses, sprayed outside of each urinal with Lysol. All that was more times than needed, but I feel, irrationally, that if I get them clean, Troy will be okay again.

Hygiene is so much better and easier than in the old days when I was a kid: "waterproof" pants in case of accidents, rubber gloves. And all this takes is love for the person you're doing it for. And … maybe … no pain for *them*. I'm *so* glad he's here.

I showed both Troy's sitter and the hospice nurse a picture of him when he was younger. I always wonder what sick people looked like when they were healthy, but a person just "can't" ask someone, "What did you look like before you were sick?"

A "spiritually interesting" thing happened this morning: Troy requested that I take the pair of underpants he's been wearing over the waterproof pants and throw them away. He said very emphatically, "Take them out of the building!" Feeling that there was a reason he asked me, I did it. When I came back he said that they needed to be thrown away because otherwise he'd be tied here. As silly as this sounds, there *may* be some truth to what he's asking that is just not believed by Christians. Different religions believe different things, and how can we tell what is "true" or not? Also, who knows what ties ghosts to a particular place?

In one hospice book I've read, there's a remark that statements of dying people should not be discounted. How can *we* tell what *they* see?

I had an old ancestor picture that I think was thrown away when I moved from Ohio that I wish I'd taken with me. Behind the picture was a letter with a passage in it about the dying person in the picture remarking about people in the corner standing and singing around a piano that was in the room.

Yes, Troy sees people, too … sometimes people he knows; sometimes not.

I took down the tray that we had set up for him in the living room and cried. It was a final admission that he really *is* dying and will not be sitting around with us any longer. I go outside to bring in the wood and look around and am reassured that the reason we're *here* is because of Troy. If we were still in Arizona, having him with us probably might not have been possible. We lived too far from just about anyplace. And, though I still don't *like* it here like I liked the Canyon, this is the place for now. I wonder when he dies, what will follow. I *do* think it's a good house, though, and peaceful.

6:08 PM

Troy: Who are you?
Me: I'm your mother.
Troy: My natural mother, or …
Me: Your natural mother.

Troy: You'll have to forgive me. I'm not feeling too well today.

6:29 PM

Troy: Do you know who I am?
Me: I call you Troy. Do you know who you are?
Troy: I call myself "Troy," but my birth name was Tim.
Do you know what (spiritual) plane we're on?
Me: The Earth plane.
Troy: What caused me to need Gatorade?
Me: You have AIDS and you're sick and your mouth was dry.

Dear God, I think, is this a repeat of November when he got worse and worse, repeating himself over and over to and from the doctor's office?! Perhaps he's on the Astral Plane, but the rest? I open two Zovirax capsules and mix them with Gatorade, hoping the problem is medical. I don't know how long he's going to live. Maybe he's going to die tomorrow, maybe not. But I *must* keep giving him medication until he dies.

Chapter 30

Saturday January 9

1:24 AM

It may be a long, awful night. I woke to Troy trying to use the urinal, which he's been doing all evening with some small results just before we got to sleep. He is still hallucinating, although he recognizes me. Is it kidney cancer? Is that why he has pressure and pain? Has he "died" (mentally)? Is that why he's hallucinating?

7:30 AM

Relief! Troy is back. He knows again *where* he is and *who* he is. I believe the medicine I gave him last night, even though it's supposed to be for herpes, has really helped … again. He still feels the need for almost constant urination. But at least he's aware of where he *really* is and knows he was having hallucinations last night. Maybe it's coincidence and the medicine *isn't* what makes him better. But I'm not taking any chances now, so I mix Gatorade and he can just continue to take it even if he doesn't particularly want it.

11:26 AM

Troy says he will die today.

5:50 PM

Troy stayed awake till about 2:45 this afternoon and then suggested we nap, which we did for about two hours. He then woke up seeing people in the room and requesting that people born on certain days leave. Then he asked for people born on Saturday. I told him I was born on a Saturday, which is true. He didn't want me to leave. He called loudly for David to come into the room. After a while since Troy seemed to be resting, I told David he might as well leave, and I would call him if Troy needed him.

Troy finally calmed down, and I emptied his urinal, washed my hands, and fixed David and me some dinner of turkey sausage and baked beans. Troy did not want any or anything else I suggested. I didn't quite know what to do. I make meals of different sorts and offer them to him, but he doesn't want them or Ensure or anything. How can I *make* him eat? I feel very helpless.

He is better, though, but *how much* better, I don't know. The hospice book says all this is normal.

I dread Wednesday because I'm scheduled to go to the unemployment office. How can I leave?

I have stomach cramps. Hopefully having eaten dinner will help, but since it was baked beans, how will I know?

6:10 PM

Troy talks softly, saying he's tired, and stares straight ahead to a point near the light on the ceiling. He'll look at me occasionally and smile. Sometimes he sleeps, eyes half-closed. This is something he's done for quite awhile. It was very startling when I first saw him do it weeks? months? ago. But he started doing it after he came here.

We held hands all morning while I sat on his bed and in the afternoon while I slept on the papasan. He doesn't want to now, though.

He looks so much like my grandmother. Because she was old and he is sick? I don't know.

6:59 PM

Troy asked me where the urinals are and I told him he had one there beside him. He said, "Oh, I goofed up again." I find his speech exceedingly touching sometimes, and I think how he has sworn about something only a few times. He reminds me, too, of a reservations agent I worked with at the Canyon. She was born in Oregon on the same day he was born in Ohio. Her daughter was born the same day as Jocelyn's last son was.

7:46 PM

I burp.

Troy: What was THAT?!
Me: It was me burping.
Troy (*He laughs lightly.*): Well, I wondered what that was!

He said a while ago that he doesn't think he'll die today after all. He was hallucinating a while before he said that and asked if hallucinating meant Death was near. I said it is possible.

We are both tired: he, because, as he has commented, he has had a big day; I, because sitting on the edge of the bed so I don't crowd him is difficult for balance.

I wish we'd bought double beds instead of twin beds to use here in this guest room that is now Troy's room. I could have lain beside him inside of sitting uncomfortably. It may mean, though, that since I am not rested maybe I will sleep tonight instead of, like usual, trying to and not being able. Will tomorrow be like today?

7:52 PM

I stood up to stretch, and when I sat down, I sat a bit on his hip. He said, "Oh." I apologized and said I'm glad he said something. I would've sat there and wondered what the bump was. He raised his eyebrows and said with a chuckle, "Yes. It's *me*!" I am so afraid I might have hurt him, but, at the same time, I try to keep it casual and not alarm either of us.

9:18 PM

Troy seems upset and tells me to call my medical friend and ask what "Trancor" means. I asked if he is dreaming and he says no and asks me again, very seriously, to call her. I do. She says she doesn't know what it is. He seems somewhat bewildered when I tell him she doesn't know.

9:58 PM

A *very* frightening story from Troy. It sounds like science fiction or something from television, but there are scientists who believe in dimensions and time travel. How can I take a chance that it's *not* true, so I decide to act like it is:

He says that between midnight and 1:30 AM tomorrow, he has to switch bodies with a girl named Susan in an experiment that has lost control. There is no way he can get out of it. They are caught in this, so I should not be surprised if he acts different. This experiment will last between eight and twelve hours. He does not know what her circumstances are, but he hopes that she is warm and has told someone on her side about this. I wonder what is *really* frightening, the thought of what might happen to him if this is real (*Can he come back? Will he be hurt?*) or the fact that I believe this might actually happen. But I know that Einstein's theory is being questioned. Scientists believe that there are more dimensions than four but can't prove them … yet. How do *we* know? What *is* reality? Will Troy laugh suddenly and say, "Ha, ha. I faked you out!"

11:00 PM

I come back from putting away the Gatorade ice cubes I've been making and find a rubber glove draped over the right side of the wastebasket, fingers on the inside of the basket, cuff on the outside. Could it be from accidentally landing there like that when I moved things around? How else could it have gotten there? But I *never, ever* intentionally leave gloves out like that because they're either dirty or they're clean. If they're dirty, I wad them up so I don't use them again by accident. If they're clean, I never would have *draped* them over the wastebasket. Then they'd be dirty and I couldn't use them. But where did it come from? How did it get in here? To my knowledge there hasn't been a glove in here for at least a couple of days! Troy's lesion is virtually healed, and I haven't needed any gloves. I've been keeping gloves in the bathroom and haven't brought any in here since I last changed his dressing. It's startling, but I decide to write it off as something I've forgotten and didn't notice earlier. But ... did Troy find it mixed in the sheets and flip it away? Is he playing tricks?

11:43 PM

Troy and I have been napping and holding hands. He kind of jerks/ pats my hand, and I ask if I can do anything. He says, "Yes. Help me." He tells me to lock the bedroom door. I pretend to, but there is no lock. Later, he asks me to unlock it. He asks for Spirit's help.

11:49 PM

He is more agitated and says we'll try next Sunday. (Is he hallucinating or dreaming?)

11:51 PM

He sleeps.
I begin reading *Transference of Consciousness at the Time of Death*, a Buddhist book.

Chapter 31

Sunday January 10 (Troy's temperature is still below 96)

8:54 AM

When I woke up I saw that Troy had removed his oxygen cannula and was holding his nose closed. It was bewildering. What was happening? Why did he feel he had to hold his nose closed? Did he think that he wasn't getting enough air and that he was holding the cannula and forcing in more oxygen? I finally *forced* him to let go of his nose and replace the cannula and then asked what he was doing. He said he was trying to relax.

It was very difficult, both because I didn't want to talk to him about dying and because the "experiment" he told me about was so weird, but finally I asked him if he thought he was going to die *today*, if he would wait until past 1:30 this afternoon. That was the time that the "experiment" was supposed to be over. He said, yes, he would. He was aware of what I was talking about. It sounds so silly and superstitious, but if I can, I will try to keep him here until then.

Christianity teaches so little of what other "pagan" religions teach and often disagrees with science, and so who is to say what can be possible? I may not be Christian, but I have grown up in a Christian society. Nonetheless, I don't want to take any chances.

It would be so easy, under the circumstances, to take it for granted that he had really died, but what if he could actually end up "stuck" someplace else? His soul would be there and he could come back to find his body gone. How can we know *positively* about things that may seem so strange to us?

So I have fixed myself some coffee and toast and have given him his medication. I rouse him from time to time to not let him slip away.

9:30 AM

I ask Troy again to wait (to die) and he says yes. I tell him that perhaps that is part of what our bargain to be together when he dies meant. He says maybe.

I've hung a magnet Buddhist-style on the end of the bed above his head to "catch his consciousness". I ask myself what is wrong with *that*?! Catholics use rosaries when they pray. I remind myself of all those years when I prayed for the living and the dead. But I'm sure that the God-consciousness or whatever is not going to hold Troy back because of the well-meaningness of an outsider someplace praying. And if it's something that is a hindrance, I'm sure God can overlook it.

Troy asks how my toast is, and I tell him it's fine. I tell him that he can have some toast, or both Gatorade liquid and ice cubes, grape Kool-Aid liquid and ice cubes, and regular water and ice cubes if he would like any. He says no.

I say, "I love you, Troy." He rubs my hand and says, "It'll be okay." He moves around but also lies with his eyes half-closed, and I can see only the white part and the bottoms of the blue. I am *sure* he will die today. I've rubbed his legs with lotion, and by helping him to *wait* comfortably for the end of the experiment, "just in case", I'm sure I'm doing all I can.

For *my own* peace of mind, though, I will use my own force of will if it's possible to not let him die before this afternoon. As I've told him many times when he's thanked me for taking care of him here and in Chicago, I'm sure he would do the same for me.

10:05 AM

I tell him it snowed last night. He says, "It's weird." (He's waited all the time he's been here for it to snow. And, now, though it's not deep or all over, it is still the heaviest it's snowed since he's been here.) "But at least it's snowed," I respond.

11:06 AM

Both his legs are up now and bent. He wants to lean them on my shoulder. "Are they too heavy?" he asks. "It's not a lot of weight?" I think to myself, "How could they *possibly* be?!"

"Are you okay?" he asks when he sees me cry.

I try to read him a card from his friend Sammie, who he also calls his sister,and begin to sob. He reads it himself and then asks if I want a hug and says that I can put my head on his chest. I do so, touching him only lightly so I am not weighing on him too heavily. He pats my shoulder. He says, "I'm afraid." I tell him to ask Spirit to help him.

11:30 AM

I tell Troy I love him and stroke his cheek. He says, "I love you, too," and asks me to kiss his cheek and turns his head to his right. I kiss him lightly. His face is stubbly from trying to grow a beard. He smiles. "I need to sleep," he says. "Okay," I tell him, "but you can't die till 1:45." (*I want to give him a grace period to make sure he's "back" from the "experiment."*) "No more experiments."

Troy: I got snaggled.
Me: Well, you've got experience now. You won't get snaggled again.

Does he *really* know who I am?

His eyes are partially closed again. No matter. "There are more things in Heaven and Earth than are explained in our philosophy" ... or something like that. If I can get him to wait a while longer, I will gladly let him go and be on his way to the world of Spirit and adventures, seeing those who have passed on to the other side.

12:45 PM

There's an hour left now before the "experiment" is finished.

I change the batteries in the tape recorder I've been using to record our talks in addition to writing down our conversations. We had long ago talked about recording during this time, and, except for one period this morning when he said the recorder light bothered him, I have been recording for about three days.

Troy: What time is it?
Me: 12:48.
Troy: Don't worry. I'm okay.

Me: I'm so sorry about asking you to wait. I just need to make sure you're all right.
Troy: What time is it again?
Me: 12:49.

I am *so* tired. But I am also so glad we talked of this time so frequently before. Did he know it would be like this but didn't want to tell me? He had said several times since coming here that he had asked to be able to experience his death in this life. He is in no apparent pain except the one day when we were waiting for the pain medicine and the nurse had asked how he felt. He's told me a lot of things, but he's never *complained*. The only discomfort is bladder pressure. He is so fortunate.

I try to meditate on goodness, light, and peace for him, but he makes deep throat sounds and I wonder if it disturbs him, so I change my mind and plan to wait to wake him.

1:00 PM

Troy: That was SOMETHING!
Me: What was that?
Troy: Moving.
Me: You've done that a lot, haven't you? *(I actually mean all the moving to different places where he's lived)*

127

Troy: It was quite an experience.

How does time pass for *him*? At 11:30, I seemed like *hours* since it had been 9:30, and now, suddenly the time, for me, has sped past.

Troy: Is this Oosala? No. *(answering his own question)* This is *your* house.
Me: Yes, it is.

1:16 PM

"Not yet," he says.
"No, not yet," I tell him.
"1:23?" he asks.
"1:25," I respond when he looks at me.
"We're waiting for *what?*"
"You can't die before 1:45." He smiles slightly and nods his head.
"Go ahead and rest," I tell him.

Die. I ask myself frequently how can I say *that* word? Then I ask, how can I *not?* Now I know why people say "gone", "passed over", "lost", when they talk about others. And I used to *laugh!* "Lost", like someone disappeared in a puff. *No*, not like *that* at all. Now I know.
It's 1:30.

1:34 PM

He looks at me. "I love you," I say and try unsuccessfully to smile. "I love you, too," he responds huskily, and I can tell he wants to cry because he sniffs. But he is too dehydrated for tears. "I'll cry for you, too," I tell him. "Thanks," he says and watches me as I let the tears run down my face, unwiped, for him.

1:37 PM

I am sitting here listening to Troy breathe, and I think of all the pictures I have of him and wonder if I really *saw* him then. We all take people for granted. I have studied his face so closely these last few months, but wonder if I *really* see him now or what I *want* to see.

I remind myself that I need to *stop* and really experience his presence while he's still here. I need to put rushing aside, and *feel* these moments. Soon, the memory of this time together will be all that I have left.

1:45 PM

When Troy was born, I looked at his face and then into his eyes. I felt a shock of recognition. It was not a *maternal* feeling of "my son", but one of *knowing* him. Now, when we look into each other's eyes, there are memories of *this* life that we've shared.

I take it for granted that he is back from his experiment. He does not say, and I am too afraid to ask what happened.

8:30 PM

Troy's friend, J, from Chicago, called just before 2:00 this afternoon, and I could not talk to him. I could not form the words, I knew I would cry. I just handed the phone to Troy when he asked who it was. J will come down this week and try to get here in the next few days.

Troy has dozed from about 5:00 PM till 7:30 when he took his two medications. He was taking more before, but with all of the pills together, there was too much stress trying to swallow. These meds seem the most critical. There are still several tablespoons to swallow to "wash down" the liquid containing the medication.

He, surprisingly, suggested that I look at his lesion. He has been too tired to lie on his side for me to apply any dressings since Friday morning. The old lesion is practically healed, but there is a dark red area *near* his tailbone, plus two *very* red marks *on* his tailbone itself and on his right hip. Potential bedsores? Kaposi's?

I take another piece of egg crate mattress and lay it between the sheet and waterproof pad to make more cushion than the one egg crate mattress he's been lying on that's under the sheet. Maybe this will help prevent further problems.

Chapter 32

Monday, January 11: b/p 80/60 at 1:10 P.M.; still not able to get a temperature

4:10 AM

Troy: Are we just waiting for me to die?

I don't answer. I pretend not to hear. This seems more of a rhetorical question than anything, and I let it pass.

I can't always tell any longer how much of my son is still with me. I can't tell if he hallucinates most of the time, though he still knows who he is, who I am, and where he is.

10:30 AM

The hospice nurse left a big wedge pillow a week or so ago for Troy to sit up with, and this morning we put it behind him. It was really an effort, and he says it may be a little too high. He's up to 5 liters on the oxygen machine. I ask him about lying down flat, and he says that all that will happen for him in that position is that he will smother. He still wants to use the pillow.

My unemployment notice on Saturday stated that I need to come in this week on Tuesday instead of Wednesday for my monthly check-in, so I've called and asked Troy's sitter if he will come over tomorrow if Troy is still okay.

1:00 PM

The hospice nurse came today and inserted a catheter to see if Troy was retaining urine. The nurse and I went into the living room so we could give him a little privacy and she could call his doctor. When we came back into the bedroom the urinal bag was almost full. Perhaps he relaxed after all the activity. He told me after she left that it was painful when the nurse was pushing on his abdomen, but now he feels much better. I didn't realize he'd had that much liquid. How could I have not understood that when he said he had bladder discomfort that his bladder was so full ?

5:00 PM

Troy does not seem to recognize me. He is agitated and wants more oxygen. I raise it back up to 5 and tell him that that is as high as it will go. He relaxes and begins to rest.

5:33 PM

I went into the living room and called Jocelyn. When I come back into the bedroom just now he knows who I am. He asks me to reposition his left leg. He has virtually ignored his right leg for quite a while now and says no when I ask him if he wants me to move it. It finally occurs to me … is it paralyzed?

"Mom," he says, "get me out of this."

6:10 PM

I've given Troy his pain medicine two and a half hours early since he says he feels bad.

He appears to know where he is again, so I ask him if it's okay if I empty the garbage. I need to get it ready for tomorrow. I've been sitting on the bed for a while with my hand on his chest. He puts his hand over mine and smiles and says yes, go ahead and get the garbage together. I start to cry, and he pats my hand. How can I change garbage at a time like this?! What will it be like tomorrow when I have to be gone all afternoon to Job Services?

We sit quietly making a hand-sandwich, mine between both of his.

"What's my oxygen on?" he asks me.

"Five. That's as high as it will go," I tell him. He nods his head and smiles strangely, knowingly.

Dying is *not* quiet. There is the rattle of the oxygen concentrator, the hiss of the oxygen, the noise of the room heater. I turn the heater off and let the room chill a little. It was too loud. I'll get a quiet one tomorrow.

Even with the oxygen level at 5 he breathes with his mouth open, though quietly. "I'm a mouth-breather," he's told me before.

The hospice nurse told me when she was here that she had not expected him to live till today.

Yes. I'm sure he's dying. His left eye closes and his right eye is partially open. I remember that only once in the hospital after he was born did he open *both* eyes at the same time.

6:32 PM

Troy's breathing changes. There are now pauses between breaths.

11:33 PM

Troy has been aware of where he is but has been hallucinating since 6:30. He has also taken down his oxygen cannula from his nose again. Even when he is aware of who and where he is he does not want to wear it. The level is set at 3.

Chapter 33

Tuesday January 12: 6/p 70/60 about noon

5:30 AM

Troy: Yesterday was a real experience. I was learning how to stay balanced in the Astral and the Physical. I was learning how to make progress. I felt the (color) blue. It was hard to maintain the blue. But I felt that to be important. The lady in red gave me a horrible, horrible time. You were the last one I saw before I left.

5:39 AM

We sing a spiritual hum together. The first time we did it today was about 4:00–4:30 AM. I feel this is significant. Before, I have sung that to him and he told me to stop after a few times. But this morning it was different; he wanted to hum longer.

Troy: I'm not doing so good. I was real dehydrated. I'm waiting for the Physical to catch up. I didn't know if I was with Love. There's a lot of love coming out of you.
Me: Out of *me*?!
Troy: Yes.
Me: That must be why we're together now.

Troy: I think we're being protected for something special.

Me: I guess we'll find out.

Troy: You have to make a journey.

Me: On the *Physical*? (I mean in comparison to what has been called "a *spiritual* journey".)

Troy: Yes.

Me: Soon?

Troy: Uh-huh.

Me: Do you where the journey will be to?

Troy: No.

How much can he tell, I wonder. Just because he's dying doesn't mean he can foresee the future. But a *journey*! That's different than a *trip*. I *should* ask, but I don't. I hope I'm not left to wonder for too long. There's so much that I *want* to ask or feel I *could* ask, but I'm afraid to.

8:20 AM

I give Troy his medicine. He stares up into the space at the ceiling overhead but drinks what I give him. I can't tell if he's aware or if he's drinking because of reflexes. So I begin to talk to him about here he is, dying; and I'm feeding him medicine, and maybe someday when we're together we'll laugh about how silly all this was. He responds clearly, "Yes."

8:30 AM

Troy: Hallelujah.

8:43 AM

I've made some phone calls. I called the sitter and told him that no matter what is determined by the State, I am *not* going in there today. I called the state job office and told the man who answered that my son is going to die soon and I will not be in. He is sympathetic and tells me to come in when I can.

I come back into the bedroom, and Troy says, plainly, "Let's hum together."

8:44 AM

Troy stops and says, "That's enough." Then, "Mom! Where's Mom?!" I tell him, "Here." He says, "Hello, Mom," once with recognition and twice mechanically. Is he trying to "hold on" like he's told me he's done before? He mumbles other things I can't understand.

8:50 AM

He seems to stop breathing. Then he continues.
My feet are cold.
Another long day?

8:53 AM

Troy says, "Death."

(It is true: fear does make a person's heart seem to stop. I can't breathe. I need to go to the bathroom.)

8:56 AM

Troy: That was nice.
Me: What was?
Troy: Seeing Light and Love. *(He mumbles something that I can't understand.)*
Me: You're a little hoarse.
Troy: Inside my throat.
Me: It's really hard, I know. You know you want to try to say something, but the words don't come out right.

9:09 AM

Troy: Oh, gosh.

9:25 AM

Troy: What have you learned?

Me: I don't know.

Troy: We need to love and to work. (*He mumbles some more that I can't hear.*) I'm still getting used to all the things that are happening.

Me: What's going on? (*For once I'm not afraid to ask. I hope to catch a glimpse of some of the things that people have talked about in near-death experiences. I will believe them if he tells me.*)

Troy: Right now, it's overcast and gloomy.

He's right; it *is* gloomy outside, here in *our* time. I don't believe he is hallucinating. I am sure he is on another plane, though, and that *his* experiences are *his* experiences, and, unfortunately, I won't be finding out about them right now. Maybe there are things that I'm not "supposed" to know yet?

9:50 AM

I sit with my left hand on Troy's chest with both of his covering mine. He seems to know that my hand is there. I can feel his heart beat.

10:05 AM

Troy: Charity is the gift of love.

Me: Charity is the gift of love? (*I repeat to make sure I've heard him correctly.*)

Troy: Yes. That's what it is. What do you think charity is?

Me: Most people seem to think that charity is giving money or furniture or clothes. I think that charity can be taking the time to do some *thing* for someone. Just like you said ... a gift of love.

10:25 AM

Troy (looking into my eyes): Are you all right?

Me: Yes. Are you?
Troy: Yeah.

11:12 AM

Troy: I was sitting here thinking of how we should come alive.
Me: Well, some of us are taught that we choose it before we're born.
Troy: We wait for him to decide what we think about.
Me: Spirit?
Troy: So it's not up to us. We're here to serve only, and we go through the process of "thought" to the life we know.
Me: I'm really glad we've got this time to spend together.
Troy: Uh-huh.

11:47 AM

I *had* thought about going to the San Francisco Zen Center later, when all this is over with, but am now considering going to stay with our friends north of here and taking my typewriter and writing our book. I can knit my rug/type/relax/grieve/walk around through the woods. I hope David doesn't mind, but it will be close, and if their kids aren't coming I can sleep late every day and stay for a week and get away for awhile.

1:00 PM

The hospice nurse has come and gone. Troy's doctor requested that the catheter be checked. She said she'll come every day now. Troy is worsening.

His sitter called a while ago and said that if there is anything he can do or errands to run, he'll be glad to do it. So I've called him back and have requested that he pick up a spiritual tape Troy would like and bring it. I've looked all over the room but can't find the one that Troy said he brought here. Maybe it will also make the sitter feel more useful, too, and a part of this even though he's known us for only a couple of weeks.

1:20 PM

Troy has abdominal pain. I hum to him while giving him his pain medicine, but he says it won't do any good right now. Burning off karma, he says. But he's very fortunate that he's not had much pain.

1:33 PM

Troy: Oh. Oh. Oh. Oh, yes. (In response to what, I don't know, since we have not been talking.)

1:41 PM

Me *(I'm concerned about giving Troy something to drink. I don't want him to have difficulty swallowing. I know his mouth must be dry. I speak clearly to him to catch his awareness.)*: I'm sorry to disturb you, Troy. I can't see what you see. I'm here on the Physical trying to make you as comfortable as possible, but maybe I should just shut up and contemplate?
Troy *(He smiles and whispers.)*: Yeah, I love you.

1:58 PM

I come in from the other room. Troy tries to hum to me, but he can't. He's hoarse. I tell him just to say the words; I'll hum for him. He says, "Yes."

2:22 PM

Troy's sitter brought the tape and has left. I wish I had asked him to stay, but I didn't. Perhaps Spirit "says" it's not the right time. Troy continues to try to hum as much as he can. I feel humanly? spiritually? selfishly? somewhat glad I didn't ask the sitter to stay, though; I'm not ready to *share* this moment ... it is *ours*.

2:48 PM

Listening to the tape and singing along with it, I am reminded of the time when I really *believed* that I heard angels singing. I was a pre-teen in Ohio. It was winter, and my parents and I lived in the country. I had gone to one of the front pastures to make angels in the snow. I heard voices singing but no words. Since I was sort of near a neighbor's house I thought perhaps it was the radio. But there was no melody. I went closer to the house and the singing stopped. I could only hear it in one portion of the pasture. I thought about what beautiful music it was. Then it stopped completely.

2:50 PM

I have gone into the bathroom, no longer afraid to leave Troy alone. This is as I visualized it would be, and he is, indeed, on the Spiritual Plane.

2:55 PM

I lean toward Troy and tell him that it's okay to go "ahead" in peace. I suddenly wonder if I had "jinxed" him in some unknown way. Did Spirit guide me?

Now I am beginning to know what dying must be about: waiting and waiting and waiting for everything to be over and finally finished even though we know we will miss the people we care most about.

3:18 PM

Can the human psyche stand only so much tension before it needs to "back off"?

I sang quietly by Troy's bed for about an hour and a half and then went into the bathroom. I went back into Troy's room and sang again for a short time, then went into the living room for a moment. I hadn't heard the phone ring, and there was a message on the answering machine from the lady who gave the tape to the sitter. I called her, telling her thanks, got my semi-frozen beer from the refrigerator, and have been sitting here, reading, writing, and listening to the tape. I feel now, with the tape, that Troy is taking care of *his* business. Perhaps a little later, I can reach the feeling of intensity of the positiveness about this I felt a while ago. Perhaps not.

4:25 PM

I have given Troy some medication. Not for pain, but the regularly scheduled maintenance kind. He "comes back" with as much force as he can muster, pushing my hands and spoon back from his face and giving me a very disgusted look. I apologize and try to explain sorrowfully that I need to try to help his *body* as long as he's here, and I don't know if that's going to be two minutes or two hours or two weeks. His eyes are open, staring.

I begin the tape again, and his eyelids start to close. As I begin to sing along with the tape again, they close completely and then half-open again as he begins to rest. A look of peace comes over his face.

I am not quite sure how disruptive I'm being with the medicine. Where does one draw the line between helping in the Earth realm and bringing him back from where he might be? How far away is he? Will my good intentions of giving him medicine impede his progress spiritually? Have I caused this (dying) to drag out longer than necessary, or will it happen in its own time? How long will I continue to interfere and continue to control? How can I tell what is helpful and what is disruptive?

7:45 PM

I have given him more pain medication and have washed up. I come back and sit down, and he looks at me. "Hello," I tell him. "Hello," he says thickly, like someone who's taken an anesthetic, and smiles. I apologize for the earlier medication incident and tell him he'll probably chew me out the next time we meet.

8:06 PM

He's obviously worsened during the day. The last time he said, "I love you," was 1:41 PM, and just a while ago it seemed to be an effort for him to just say hello.

Am I doing enough for him? Does he need more liquid? I'll give him more "regular" medication at 8:30 and more Gatorade. I know he's close to death, but *how close*? Do I continue to pour Gatorade down his throat or leave him alone? *How can I tell*? He did not respond to any of my questions earlier. I asked him if he wanted anything, and if he did, maybe he could blink his eyes. He continued to look at me with no response. The "Hello" was a surprise.

8:43 PM

I turn the religious tape to the other side and feel a real need to call some of his friends. I had intended to call them only after he dies but really feel I *need* to call right now.

10:00 PM

I won't be turning the tape back over. It has only twenty minutes a side, and I need to get some sleep. Perhaps Troy will live another night. He will wake me if he needs me. I kiss his forehead. He is sweating, something he has not done for quite a while. He had put his arms under the covers earlier. Perhaps he is hot. I turn down the blanket and take out his arms.

10:23 PM

I worry. Maybe Troy's cold. I put his arms back under the blanket.

10:25 PM

Perhaps the weight of the blanket is too much and he won't be able to take out his arms if the blankets are too heavy. I can imagine him telling me that I'm buzzing around too fast again and decide to leave him alone and rest. I move back to my papasan and try to sleep.

Chapter 34

Wednesday January 13

1:45 AM

I hear Troy say the word *"Air!"* and wake up to see him flailing his arms. I ask him what's wrong. Is it pain? I turn his oxygen machine up to 4. He calms down somewhat but is still agitated. He is inhaling with tiny breaths and exhaling loudly. If it were breathing distress, wouldn't he be inhaling loudly and gasping for breath?

Is his body trying to help his soul leave?

I call the hospice nurse line, and the nurse calls back. I tell her what is going on. She tells me something I don't remember. I tell her that I have tried giving him some Gatorade on a sponge and wetting his mouth to take medication, but he seems to be having a hard time swallowing.

What can I do so that I won't choke him? She suggests putting the crushed pain medication in jelly and putting it in the corner of his mouth. I ask her to stay on the phone with me while I do it and keep mumbling to her as I go into the kitchen to make it.

I take the jelly/medicine combination into the bedroom and try giving him some.

He is still breathing in large exhales, and I put the phone to his face, asking the nurse to listen to him. I see him swallow and stop. His mouth opens and shuts, and his jaws clamp together. I take his pulse. I can no longer feel his heart beat.

"I think he's died," I tell her.

"*He can still hear you!*" she says. "I'm getting ready to come over. Call me back." And she hangs up.

I realize *finally* that he is still here spiritually and I need to help him!!! I turn the tape back on and lean forward to his ear. "I love you. Find Spirit. Find the Blue. Blessings be." I begin to hum for him.

His face has been turned to his right, and he turns now to face me. We look into each other's eyes, he smiles at me, and I actually see his spirit fading from his gaze. His soul has left his body, and he slumps to his left. The clock says 2:01.

****

It is 2:28 AM, and I keep looking at him, expecting him to turn back to me and smile and say, "Surprise. Still here." It's absurd. I feel foolish. But I still won't admit that he's gone.

I turn off the oxygen. There is nothing I can do except let the tape play. His spirit may be still here, or perhaps he's left to go on ahead. I call back the nurse and she says she's on the way to us. I tell David that Troy has died.

Even though I know that when Hospice has been involved with a dying patient and the police do not come to the scene, I still move the furniture back out of the way to make more room. I continue to play the tape and wonder if Troy is still here with me or off with friends and family who are welcoming him back to the Spirit Plane. There seems no need to talk to him right now.

I begin to pace in the small area of the room and up and down the hall, back and forth between the bedroom and the living room.

This is a bad dream. Everything is not really over. I think that I will wake up before long and he will be well again … or alive. But I know he will not.

I walk in and out of the room, turning the tape over when I realize it has stopped playing. I don't feel sorry, only sad. There is tension and anticipation of waiting for the funeral home people to arrive.

The hospice nurse arrives and says she would like to clean Troy's body. She washes his face and calls the funeral home to come and take his body away.

Two young men with the hearse arrive what seems to be a short time later. Everything is quiet and very well-handled. No tromping through the house saying, "What's going on here?!" But they are not the police. They wheel the gurney into the bedroom while I stand in the hall so I won't get in their way.

They close the door. Then they open it. The nurse asks if I want to come in. "Yes, please," I tell her. "It will help my grieving process to realize he's gone. And besides, Troy and I decided to go through the *whole thing* together." Am I intellectualizing this to protect myself?

I watch as one of the men lifts Troy's body from the bed and carries him to the gurney. I crawl over the bed and stand by his shoulder and touch his cheek. "Goodbye, Troy," I tell him. "I love you."

We all walk together to the front door in a small procession down the short hall. The attendants pull the white body bag up to cover Troy's face. I wonder how he will stay warm. It is cold outside. How will he breathe with his face covered? I start to sag without knowing it until David grabs me to hold me up.

I *need* to see this. I was there when he was born, and now that he has died, I need to realize it and deal with it. I can meet him spiritually, but it's his *body* that I have looked at over the years, and I need to know that he has left it.

The attendants push the gurney into the hearse, and they drive away. The nurse follows.

It is quiet. There are only David and me in the house now.

We sit in the living room and talk. I get up periodically and turn the tape over, but finally it is 5:00 AM. As I go toward the bedroom I know there is no need to play it is again, but I say out loud, "I will play it one more time," and leave the room. I feel that the room is empty now.

David is willing to stay home, but I tell him that although it is kind of him to say that he'll do that, it is not necessary. I don't know what he could do. I would feel more comfortable alone.

Troy's "visit" is over. He will come back, I'm sure, at times, if he won't become "attached" to the house. But I think that the tape has helped his spirit to go on. I feel strangely calm and am, again, thankful that we had been able to be together these last months. If we had not been, I do not know if I could handle the grief. But because of the time we could spend together, there is no grief, only an unfamiliar *emptiness* that I haven't felt before.

I feel bad for people whose loved ones die suddenly and they have no way to tell them that they will miss them.

As odd as it sounds, I can begin to start to understand the Buddhist story of the man who was celebrating and laughing when his wife died. He knew that finally she was all right. Like hers, Troy's sickness is over.

7:33 AM

Looking out the front door, I decide that I will keep Troy's urn in the house rather than bury it under a tree. He's not a "cow person," he told me once when I was pointing out a neighbor's cows in a field. Our neighbor may want to turn his cows out into our yard.

I look out the window in the front door and see a big rabbit run south across our parking area in front of me. I think how silly it is, but wonder if it's a message from Troy. Except for Cookie, the small ceramic dragon he bought me when he was visiting us in August, he has given me a lot of rabbit figures. But who knows; "strange things" happen, and I like to think the rabbit is a remembrance from him. I turn away from the door to call some of his friends before they leave for work.

11:34 AM

Sherry, his friend from Chicago, told me when I called her earlier that she had had a dream of the three of us and some others of his friends in a circle in what she thought is my front yard. That was nice to hear because it helps me believe he's okay. I'm glad she told me.

Sammie, his "sister" in California, told me when I called her that she had considered calling me earlier to tell me about her experience. About midnight, her (Pacific) time and 2:00 AM our time when Troy was dying, she was talking to a friend in Hawaii who said suddenly, "Troy is here." Sammie said that about 3:00 AM her time (I still hadn't called her yet) she was sitting on her couch since she couldn't sleep and felt a hand on hers. She stood up and felt a hug. These are things that I am sure some people will feel are made up, but who knows. I will believe them. Sammie and her friend did not know at those times that Troy had died.

I know I will miss him desperately at times and will want to hear him say, "I love you," *just once more*, but I know I will now have to open myself up and visit with him interiorally, spiritually.

****

Epilogue

This book is to my son and friend, and to all the people in the world who have loved and been loved throughout history.

Writing this is a contribution that Troy and I wanted to make to other people, like us, whose family members and loved ones were dying, no matter what the disease. This is something we discussed ever since he was diagnosed with AIDS.

Why a book about *dying*, a story of someone loved being forever separated from those left behind? Why not write something happier, cheerful, more positive?

Perhaps because, as I've said, for several years and after many discussions, Troy decided that he would like *his* contribution to the stream of life to be a record of his passing, a contribution to others who would be able to spend last days with those they love. It would be a record that would help others understand that they, too, can spend close hours together that will make the separation easier.

We tried tape recording in the hospital and the first days at home but gave it up after finding out that we were talking more to the machine than to each other. So the early days together are the memories and "summings up" that I wrote in my diary.

Then we began to feel that it was more appropriate to write down conversations as they occurred.

During Troy's final three or four days of life, we used a voice-activated recorder, except when he was dying. We had turned the recorder off earlier when we had gone to sleep.

I have not listened to more than only a few minutes of those tapes. Perhaps someday.

The tapes and this written record remain an encouragement, both my son and I hope, to those people who would like to truly share the ending of their lives together.

It is odd how we expect the people that we love to be with us forever. Selfishly, we want to keep them near us no matter how sick they may be or how ready they are to "go ahead".

To me, Troy has never died. He was able to move to different cities when he was living, so now I try to imagine him being just a phone call away.

I sing "Happy Birthday" to him each year.

Wouldn't it be nice, I think, that when we die, that the people we love might sing "Happy Birthday" to us, too.

Fly, my son. Fly away. Visit the inner spiritual worlds. Meet those who have gone on. Share your experiences. Progress spiritually.

I love you.

May the blessings be.

www.ingramcontent.com/pod-product-compliance
Lightning Source LLC
Chambersburg PA
CBHW020438290526
45785CB00002B/913